COLOR ATLAS
DERMATOLOGY

THIRD EDITION

Gary White MD

Associate Clinical Professor
University of California, San Diego, California, USA

 Mosby

Edinburgh London New York Oxford Philadelphia St Louis Sydney Toronto 2004

MOSBY
ELSEVIER
An imprint of Elsevier Limited

Third edition 2004
 Reprinted 2004 (twice), 2007

ISBN 13: 978 07234 3298 2
ISBN 10: 0 7234 3298 8

British Library Cataloguing in Publication Data
A catalogue record for this book is available from the British Library

Library of Congress Cataloging in Publication Data
A catalog record for this book is available from the Library of Congress

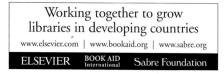

ELSEVIER your source for books, journals and multimedia in the health sciences
www.elsevierhealth.com

Working together to grow libraries in developing countries
www.elsevier.com | www.bookaid.org | www.sabre.org
ELSEVIER   BOOK AID International   Sabre Foundation

The Publisher's policy is to use paper manufactured from sustainable forests

Printed in Spain

CONTENTS

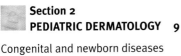

Section 1
MORPHOLOGY

MORPHOLOGY

MORPHOLOGIC AND DESCRIPTIVE TERMINOLOGY

The importance of using the correct terms when describing a dermatologic condition cannot be over-emphasized. To the uninitiated, every rash is 'maculopapular'. The majority of dermatologic diseases, however, are not. In addition to its morphology, a lesion's color, number, configuration, and distribution are of vital importance. Much of the process of learning dermatology involves learning its language. The following pages contain illustrations of some of these terms.

MORPHOLOGIC TERMS (see pages 4–7)

Macule/patch   A color change of the skin only. There is no elevation, induration, or scale. If you close your eyes and feel only, you cannot tell it is there. The difference between a macule and a patch is one of size, i.e. a patch is greater than 1 cm in diameter.

Papule/nodule   A raised spot on the surface of skin. The difference between a papule and a nodule is one of size, i.e. a nodule is greater than 5 mm. The word tumor is sometimes used to describe a large nodule (see **Figure ii**).

Plaque   A raised uniform thickening of a portion of the skin with a well-defined edge and a flat or rough surface (see **Figure iii**).

Vesicle/bulla   A fluid-filled blister. The term vesicle is used if the lesion is less than 5 mm, and the term bulla is used if the lesion is greater than 5 mm (see **Figure iv**).

Pustule   A bleb of skin filled with pus.

Fissure   A crack or split in the epidermis (see **Figure v**).

Erosion   An area of partial loss of the epidermis (see **Figure vi**).

Ulcer   An area of total loss of the epidermis (see **Figure vii**).

Atrophy/lipoatrophy   Atrophy is loss of thickness or substance of the epidermis or dermis. Lipoatrophy is loss of the subcutaneous fat.

Wheal   A transient pink plaque caused by edema of the skin, usually restricted to describing urticaria.

Petechia/purpura   Purple discoloration of the skin caused by the extravasation of blood. A lesion less than 5 mm is a petechia, one greater than 5 mm is called purpura.

Papulosquamous   This term is used to describe conditions that manifest themselves as papules or plaques with scale, e.g. psoriasis, pityriasis rosea, and secondary syphilis.

Eczematous   This term is used to describe inflammatory conditions of the skin that appear erythematous and scaly with ill-defined borders, e.g. atopic dermatitis, irritant dermatitis, etc.

Necrosis   Death of the skin.

SURFACE CHANGES (see pages 7–8)

Scaly   Covered by flakes of flat horny cells loosened from the horny layer (i.e. the stratum corneum) (see **Figure viii**).

Wet/oozing   The water barrier of the skin has been damaged and there is enough flow of fluid from below to keep the surface of the lesion wet.

Crusted   Usually refers to dried serum, but sometimes the term is applied to a thick mass of horny cells or to a mixture of both (see **Figure ix**).

Excoriated   This term means that the lesion has been scratched. The presence of linear erosions or scabs indicates this fact. Old excoriations may turn into linear white scars.

Lichenified   Thickening of the epidermis with an exaggeration of normal skin lines (see **Figure x**). This change occurs almost exclusively after chronic rubbing.

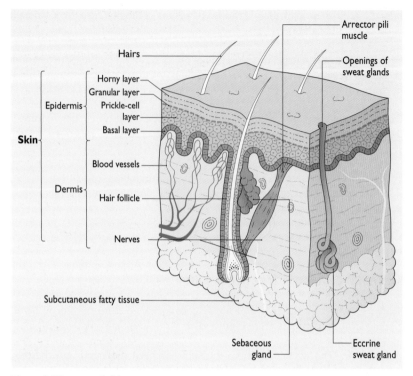

Arrector pili muscle

Hairs

Openings of sweat glands

Horny layer
Granular layer
Epidermis — Prickle-cell layer
Basal layer

Skin

Blood vessels

Dermis — Hair follicle

Nerves

Subcutaneous fatty tissue

Sebaceous gland

Eccrine sweat gland

Figure i. Diagram of skin structure.

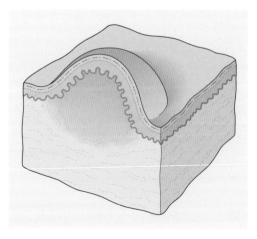

Figure ii. Papule/nodule: a raised spot on the surface of skin. The difference between a papule and a nodule is one of size, i.e. a nodule is greater than 5 mm. The word tumor is sometimes used to describe a large nodule.

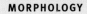

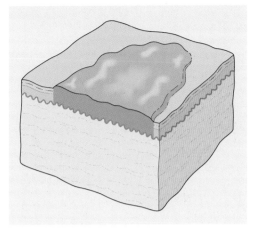

Figure iii. Plaque: a raised uniform thickening of a portion of the skin with a well-defined edge and a flat or rough surface.

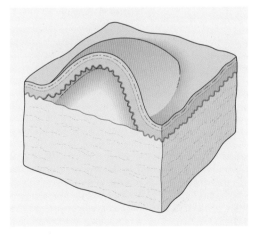

Figure iv. Vesicle/bulla: a fluid-filled blister. The term vesicle is used if the lesion is less than 5 mm, and the term bulla is used if the lesion is greater than 5 mm.

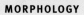
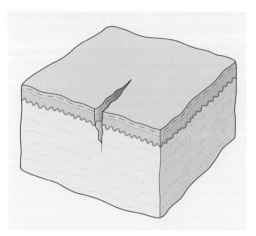

Figure v. Fissure: a crack or split in the epidermis.

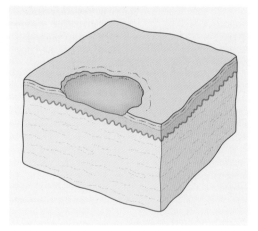

Figure vi. Erosion: an area of partial loss of the epidermis.

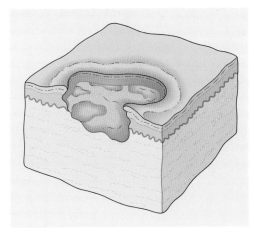

Figure vii. Ulcer: an area of total loss of the epidermis.

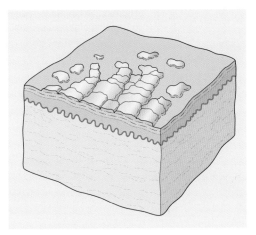

Figure viii. Scaly: covered by flakes of flat horny cells loosened from the horny layer (i.e. the stratum corneum).

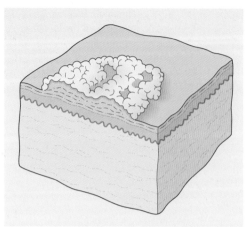

Figure ix. Crusted: usually refers to dried serum, but sometimes the term is applied to a thick mass of horny cells or to a mixture of both.

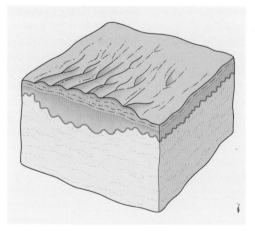

Figure x. Lichenified: thickening of the epidermis with an exaggeration of normal skin lines.

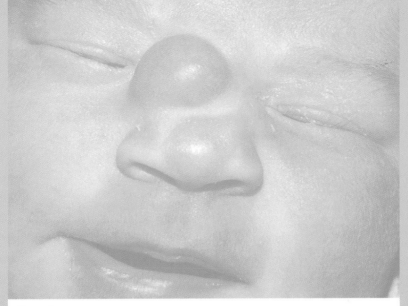

Section 2
PEDIATRIC DERMATOLOGY

CONGENITAL AND NEWBORN DISEASES

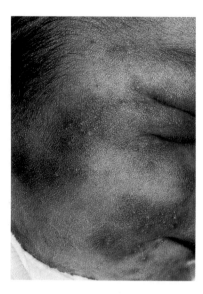

Figure 1. Erythema toxicum is a benign and transient condition typical of healthy newborns. The etiology is unknown. It presents as an erythematous patch, 1–3 cm in diameter, with a central papulopustule. Eosinophils are predominant in the sterile pustules and in dermal lesions. It must be distinguished from other more serious causes of pustular lesions, e.g. impetigo, scabies, herpes, etc. Gram or Giemsa stain and potassium hydroxide examination (see **Figure 321**) are helpful in establishing the diagnosis.

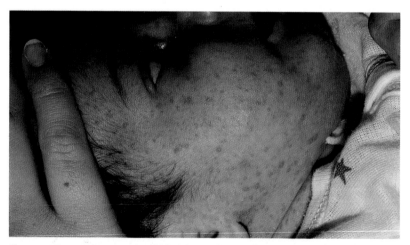

Figure 2. Neonatal acne. A mild facial acneiform eruption is common in the first month of life. The presence of the fungus *Malassezia* species has been associated, but further studies are needed to prove this agent is causative. Patients present with facial papules and pustules.

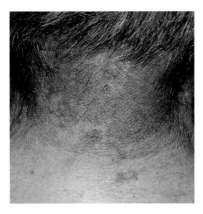

Figure 3. Erythema nuchae, salmon patch, and port wine stain are similar flat, congenital, vascular lesions which present as pink or red patches. The term stain is used because the skin is not altered in any way other than in color. Erythema nuchae by definition occurs on the nape of an infant. It is benign and extremely common. The lesion may spontaneously involute, or persist throughout life as shown here.

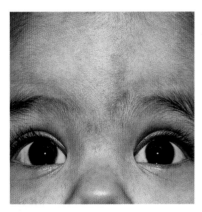

Figure 4. Salmon patch is defined as a vascular blanching red patch or streak across the forehead and/or glabella in a newborn infant. In contrast to a port wine stain, the salmon patch is usually lighter in color, not dermatomally distributed, and will spontaneously involute.

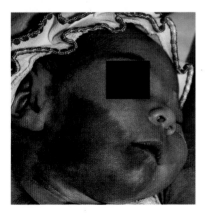

Figure 5. Port wine stain is a congenital, fixed, flat, red or pink patch. It may occur as an isolated finding or in association with several syndromes. The distribution often follows a dermatome, and the dermatome involved is key in determining management. Facial port wine stains involving V1 may be associated with ocular abnormalities (e.g. glaucoma, choroidal angioma) with or without Sturge–Weber syndrome (see **Figure 6**). The child shown here with a port wine stain of V3 is at risk for neither. Cosmesis is the main concern.

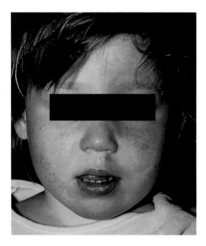

Figure 6. Sturge–Weber syndrome is a non-inherited disorder that combines a facial port wine stain involving the V1 dermatome (forehead, upper and lower eyelid, and side of the nose), seizures, and ipsilateral leptomeningial angiomatosis. If the port wine stain is in the V2 (upper lip, cheek) and/or V3 (lower lip, chin, jawline, ear and preauricular) dermatome without involvement of V1, there is no need to rule out Sturge–Weber syndrome. Involvement of all three—V1, V2, and V3—significantly increases the risk of Sturge–Weber syndrome (as shown here).

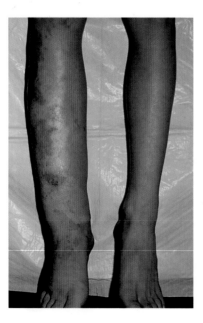

Figure 7. Klippel–Trenaunay syndrome is a disorder that combines a congenital nevus flammeus (also known as port wine stain) and ipsilateral hypertrophy of the bones and/or soft tissue. An extremity is usually affected. Varicose veins develop later in the majority and can cause pain and swelling. Other potential complications include hematochezia, hematuria, cellulitis, and thrombophlebitis. A variety of associated serious congenital malformations have been reported. (Courtesy of Michael O Murphy, MD.)

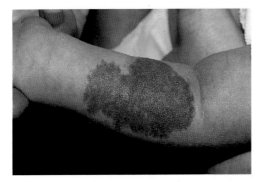

Figure 8. Capillary hemangioma. Capillary hemangiomas are benign vascular proliferations that occur more commonly in preterm infants and females (female to male ratio is 3:1). At birth they may present as: a barely visible, white, anemic stain; a faint, telangiectatic lesion; a flat, red patch, as shown here; a blue spot mimicking a bruise; or, rarely, a full grown hemangioma. Other terms include infantile hemangioma and, simply, hemangioma.

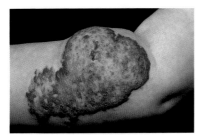

Figure 9. Capillary hemangioma. Capillary hemangiomas are distinguished from vascular malformations (e.g. port wine stain, arteriovenous malformation) by the fact that they proliferate, typically during the first 3–9 months of life. This picture shows the same child as in **Figure 8** but was taken several weeks later. The diagnosis of a capillary hemangioma is usually made clinically, but lesions that are excessively firm deserve careful evaluation and possibly biopsy, as tumors such as rhabdomyosarcomas, infantile myofibromatosis, and nasal gliomas (see **Figure 15**) can resemble hemangiomas.

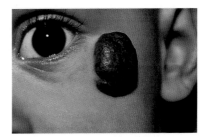

Figure 10. Capillary hemangioma, periocular. In addition to being cosmetically disfiguring, periocular capillary hemangiomas have the potential to cause serious ocular complications such as amblyopia, strabismus, proptosis, and optic atrophy. If this hemangioma were to grow to the point that it obstructed vision, treatment would be mandatory.

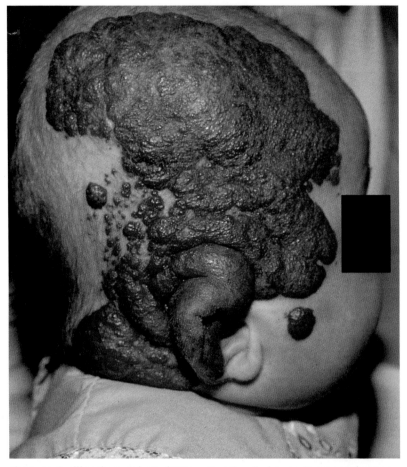

Figure 11. Capillary hemangioma, large. Occasionally, hemangiomas may become rather large and disfiguring. Potential complications include ulceration, bleeding, infection, and high output cardiac failure. Large facial hemangiomas may be associated with brain malformations, e.g. the Dandy–Walker malformation. Hemangiomas are a feature of a syndrome to which the term PHACE has been applied (**p**osterior fossa malformations, **h**emangiomas, **a**rterial anomalies, **c**oarctation of the aorta, and **c**ardiac defects and **e**ye abnormalites). Hemangiomas overlying the anterior neck may be associated with airway involvement and obstruction. A plaque-like hemangioma spanning the midline of the sacrum may be associated with an underlying tethered spinal cord. (Courtesy of Michael O Murphy, MD.)

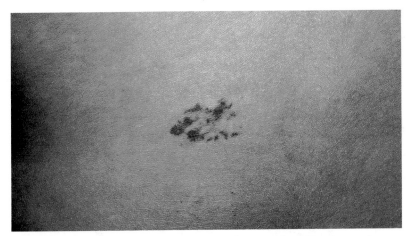

Figure 12. Capillary hemangioma, involuting. If untreated, capillary hemangiomas may spontaneously involute, leaving normal skin, slight redness, telangiectasia, wrinkling and/or sagging. Such spontaneous resolution occurs in 50% of patients by 5 years and 70% by 7 years. The site of a previous hemangioma in this 3-year-old child shows telangiectasia and slight hypopigmentation.

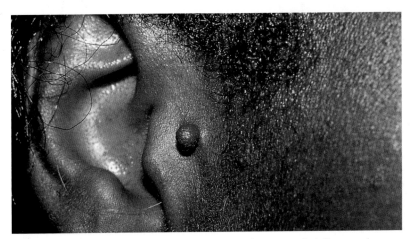

Figure 13. Accessory tragus. The accessory tragus is a congenital, firm papule or multilobular nodule occurring in the preauricular area and occurs in roughly 0.5% of children. The lesion may consist of only skin or skin and cartilage. It is usually solitary, but may occasionally be bilateral or familial. The vast majority of lesions are isolated, but other abnormalities of the first and second branchial arch may rarely occur, e.g. oculoauriculovertebral syndrome (Goldenhar syndrome).

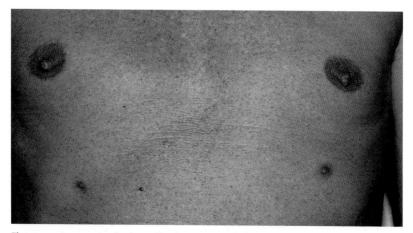

Figure 14. Accessory nipple. Also known as polythelia, the accessory nipple appears as a small, brown papule which may resemble a nipple, along the milk line that stretches from the axilla through the normal nipple to the groin. One, two (as shown), or more may occur. If two occur, they often appear on opposite sides at the same level. There is an equal sex and side incidence. The vast majority of lesions are isolated, but rare cases of associated abnormalities (e.g. renal) have been reported.

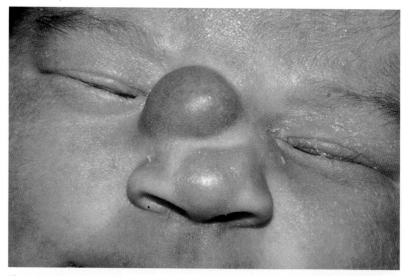

Figure 15. Nasal glioma is a congenital benign tumor of the nasal region containing neural tissue. There is no connection with the central nervous system, in contrast to a nasal encephalocele. A congenital, firm, non-transilluminating, blue or red nodule just lateral to the nasal root is characteristic. It does not change size or shape as a result of crying or straining, nor does it distend with jugular vein compression. Vascular lesions, nasal encephaloceles, and dermoid cysts are in the differential diagnosis. Imaging of the central nervous system is mandatory prior to biopsy or removal.

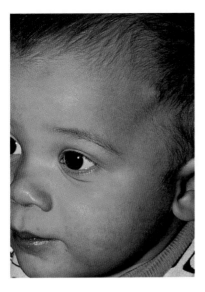

Figure 16. Dermoid cyst is a common benign tumor mainly observed in the head and neck area. It results from a sequestration of cutaneous elements along embryonic lines of fusion. A firm or rubbery, painless nodule, present congenitally or noticed in the first 2 decades of life, is characteristic. It tends to occur on the scalp and face, especially at the lateral third of the eyebrow, but may also occur in the nasal area, oral cavity, or lateral neck. An underlying sinus may be present and extend to the scalp, the skull, the extradural space, or within the subarachnoid space. This child's dermoid cyst is seen above the temple along the hairline.

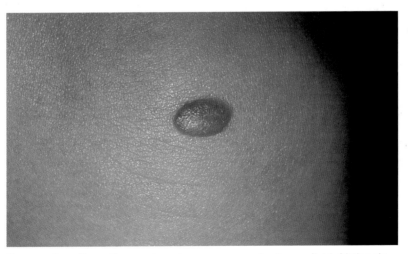

Figure 17. Juvenile xanthogranuloma is an uncommon, benign, pediatric histiocytic tumor that usually presents in the skin, but may occasionally occur in the eye, soft tissue, or viscera. A yellowish-red papulonodule in a newborn or young child is characteristic, although adults may be affected. Multiple lesions may occur.

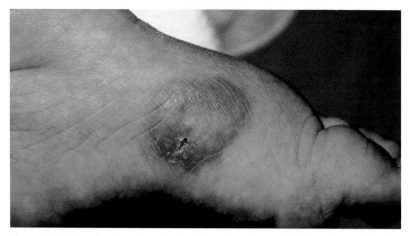

Figure 18. Solitary mastocytoma is a benign tumor that results from the accumulation of mast cells in the skin. It may be present at birth or develop within the first few weeks of life. It may have an orange-peel surface and will urticate (Darier's sign) or even blister upon stroking. Note the reddish-orange color. (See also **Figures 103–105**.)

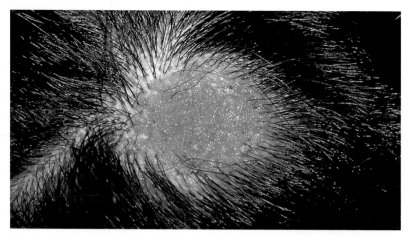

Figure 19. Nevus sebaceous is a congenital hamartoma of sebaceous glands. A round or oval, red to yellow, smooth plaque on the scalp at birth is characteristic. The face is the second most commonly affected site. A rare type of diffuse epidermal nevus may exhibit sebaceous differentiation.

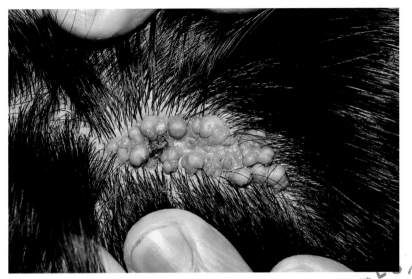

Figure 20. Nevus sebaceous at puberty. At puberty, under hormonal influence, the nevus sebaceous may become verrucous or studded with multiple papules—like a mulberry.

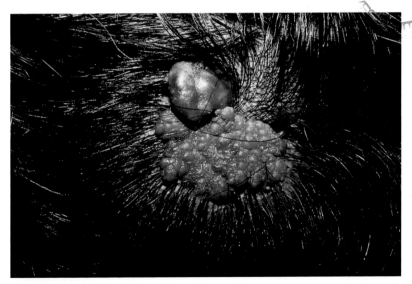

Figure 21. Basal cell carcinoma arising in a nevus sebaceous. Many appendageal neoplasms—both benign and malignant—may develop within the nevus sebaceous. Syringocystadenoma papilliferum or basal cell carcinoma are the most common. A basal cell carcinoma developed in this nevus sebaceous. (Courtesy of Michael O Murphy, MD)

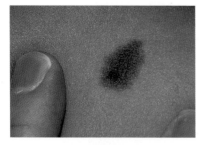

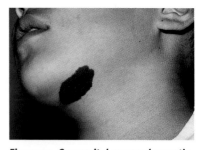

Figure 22. Congenital nevomelanocytic nevus, small. This lesion results from a congenital deposition of nevomelanocytic cells. Melanoma can develop, but such an event is rare for small congenital nevi (i.e. those with diameter <1.5 cm). Any focal change should be considered for biopsy. The new pigmented area in this lesion was benign.

Figure 23. Congenital nevomelanocytic nevus, medium. The risk of melanoma is still low for medium-sized lesions (>1.5 cm but <20 cm). Many hairs may be present as illustrated in this small to medium lesion.

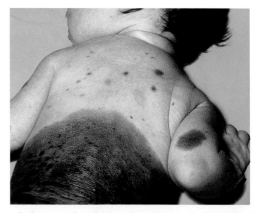

Figure 24. Congenital nevomelanocytic nevus, giant. An extensive (>20 cm), black, verrucous, congenital nevus covering a large area of the body—commonly including the low back and thighs—is characteristic. Multiple smaller, satellite lesions may be scattered over the rest of the skin and even mucous membranes (and are seen in this child on the upper back and arms). The incidence of developing melanoma is significant, with most estimates between 2% and 6%. Melanoma typically does not develop in satellite lesions—only in the main pigmented area. Unfortunately, this infant died of melanoma. Neurocutaneous melanosis is the combination of melanocytes of the skin and central nervous system. It is associated most commonly with giant congenital melanocytic nevi, in particular those on the scalp or in a posterior axial location that are accompanied by satellite nevi. (Courtesy of O Dale Collins III, MD.)

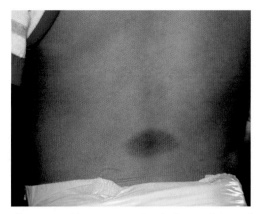

Figure 25. Mongolian spot.   The presence of melanin-containing cells within the dermis (dermal melanocytosis) occurs in a variety of nevi, usually categorized by their location. The Mongolian spot occurs over the low back and sacrum, the Nevus of Ota (**Figure 26**) on the face, and the Nevus of Ito on the back. The deeper localization of the pigment gives the skin a bluish hue as a result of the Tyndall effect. The Mongolian spot is most common in Asians, then dark-skinned peoples and least commonly in Caucasians. The typical lesion occurs over the sacrum and tends to fade over time. Congenital blue patches occurring away from the sacrum often persist and are sometimes called aberrant Mongolian spots.

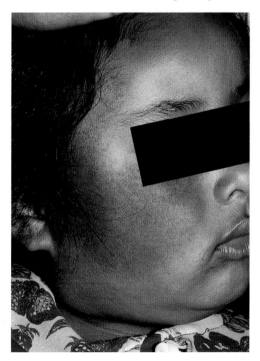

Figure 26. Nevus of Ota is a unilateral, congenital, blue-black pigmentation in the distribution of the trigeminal nerve (predominantly V1 and V2, as shown here). Pigmentation may also be found in the oral mucosa, sclera and tympanic membrane. Onset is at birth or soon after in approximately half of cases. Nearly all lesions develop by age 30 years. Dark-skinned and Asian patients are more commonly affected, and there is a female predominance.

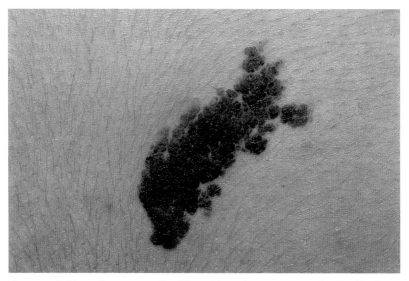

Figure 27. Epidermal nevus, small.   The epidermal nevus represents a localized hyperplasia of epidermal elements. The color may be brown, pink or white and the size may range from small, as here, to very extensive. The widely distributed type may be associated with systemic abnormalities of the musculoskeletal, ocular, and neurological systems (known as the epidermal nevus syndrome).

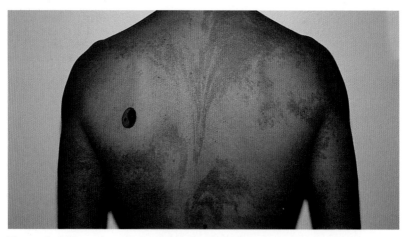

Figure 28. Epidermal nevus, large (a tattoo is also seen over the left scapula). Alfred Blaschko, a private practitioner of dermatology in Berlin, transposed the linear pattern of the skin lesions of more than 140 patients onto dolls and statues. His composite diagram has since been referred to as Blaschko's lines. They are thought to result from the dorsoventral outgrowths of two different cell populations during early embryogenesis. Many congenital skin diseases, including epidermal nevi, may be distributed according to its pattern.

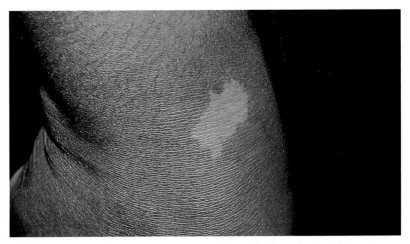

Figure 29. Nevus depigmentosus is a congenital, stable, hypopigmented macule or patch located randomly, segmentally, linearly, or in a whorled fashion. Melanocytes are present histologically but do not produce the usual amount of melanin. Wood's light accentuates the lesion. Because some pigment is present, perhaps a more accurate name is nevus hypopigmentosus. Over 90% of lesions present before 3 years of age. When it is systematized, it is indistinguishable from hypomelanosis of Ito.

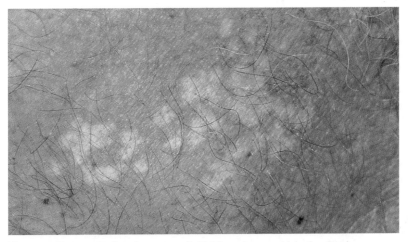

Figure 30. Nevus anemicus is a congenital birthmark caused by a localized, permanent vasoconstriction of blood vessels. The relative lack of blood gives it a whitish color. The defect appears to be a result of increased local sensitivity to catecholamines. If the skin is grafted to another site, it retains its vasoconstriction, thus implying that the blood vessels themselves have an increased sensitivity to catecholamines as opposed to increased sympathetic stimulation. There is no alteration of pigment, and its border may thus be obliterated for several seconds by rubbing a finger across it. Rarely, the nevus anemicus may be associated with certain genodermatoses, including neurofibromatosis and phakomatosis pigmentovascularis.

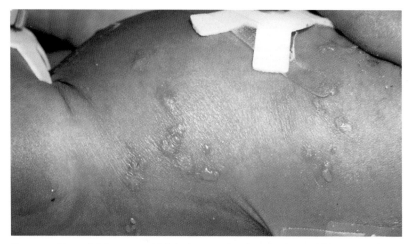

Figure 31. Neonatal herpes. A blistering eruption in a newborn which represents herpes simplex infection is a medical emergency. Transmission may have occurred transplacentally or via the birth canal. Systemic involvement can include encephalitis, pneumonia, and hepatitis. (Courtesy of Michael O Murphy, MD.)

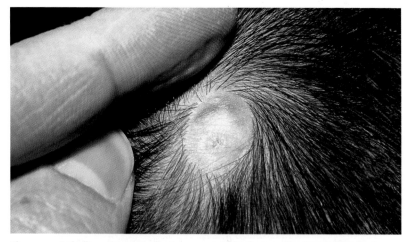

Figure 32. Aplasia cutis congenita is a congenital, circumscribed area of alopecia and scarring typically occurring on the scalp. Small lesions are usually isolated findings, but larger lesions may be associated with various abnormalities, e.g. trisomies (e.g. 10, 13), underlying skull defects and distal limb abnormalities (Adams–Oliver syndrome), and epidermolysis bullosa. The presence of dense hair at the periphery (hair collar sign) should raise the possibility of a more significant defect (e.g. rudimentary meningocele).

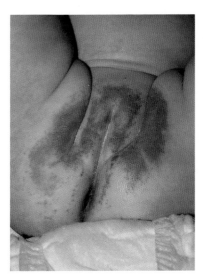

Figure 33. Diaper dermatitis.
The diaper area is red and edematous but the flexures are usually spared (in contrast to seborrheic dermatitis, **Figure 35**) in diaper dermatitis. This is an irritant dermatitis from the stool and urine and is worsened by maceration and friction. A bout of diarrhea may bring on or exacerbate the condition.

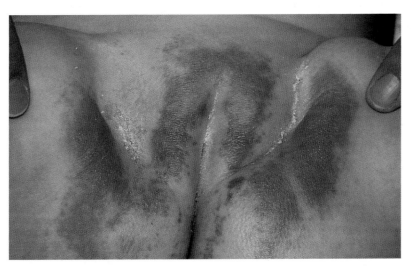

Figure 34. Diaper dermatitis. Note the characteristic sparing of the flexures.

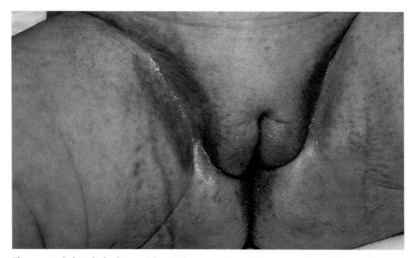

Figure 35. Seborrheic dermatitis, groin.   In seborrheic dermatitis of infants, the groin is red and scaly, with prominent involvement of the flexures (in contrast to diaper dermatitis, **Figures 33** and **34**). The scalp is frequently red and scaly. The onset is from 2 weeks to 6 months.

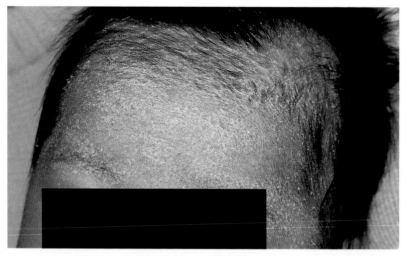

Figure 36. Seborrheic dermatitis, cradle cap.   Seborrheic dermatitis in the infant commonly affects the scalp. When it does, the term cradle cap is used. Note the presence of abundant scale in the scalp.

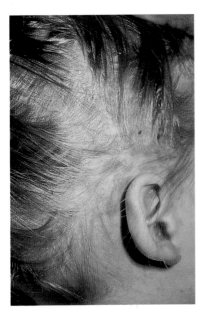

Figure 37. Langerhans' cell histiocytosis, scalp. Langerhans' cell histiocytosis (formerly called histiocytosis X) is a disorder of unknown etiology that gives rise to clonal expansion of Langerhans'-like cells or their precursors. Classically, Langerhans' cell histiocytosis has been separated into Letterer–Siwe disease (infants, aggressive, internal involvement), Hand–Schüller–Christian disease (children, bony defects especially of the skull, diabetes insipidus, and exophthalmos) and eosinophilic granuloma (children and adults, granulomas of the skin and bones, benign, chronic). Electron microscopy shows a significant number of the cells to contain Birbeck granules, which resemble racquets. The infant with Langerhans' cell histiocytosis may present with a red, scaly, seborrheic-dermatitis-like rash of the scalp and flexures. (Courtesy of Michael O Murphy, MD.)

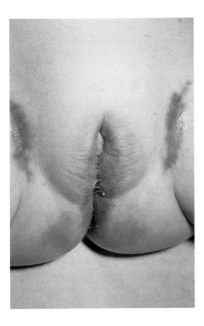

Figure 38. Langerhans' cell histiocytosis, groin. A red, scaly intertrigo-like rash of the groin is characteristic. (Courtesy of Michael O Murphy, MD.)

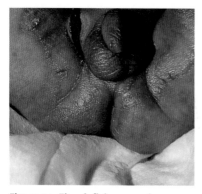

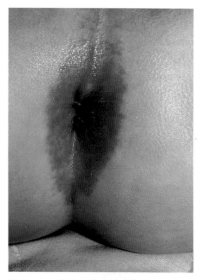

Figure 39. Zinc deficiency, groin.
A pustular, bullous, and erosive eruption may develop periorally, perianally, acrally, and in the genital region in an infant with deficient zinc intake. Infants receiving artificial feeding, or breast-fed infants whose mother's milk is deficient in zinc, may be affected. Other diseases that may cause a similar rash include acrodermatitis enteropathica, cystic fibrosis, treated maple syrup urine disease, inborn errors of biotin metabolism, ornithine transcarbamylase deficiency, and neonatal citrullinemia. (Courtesy of James Steger, MD.)

Figure 40. Perianal cellulitis is a dermatitis of the perianal skin caused by group A beta-hemolytic streptococci. Clinically, one sees a well-demarcated perianal erythema, which may be accompanied by itching, bleeding, and painful defecation. Children aged 7 months to 8 years are most commonly affected.

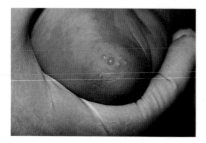

Figure 41. Infantile acropustulosis is a rare, benign, and transient pustular dermatosis seen in infants and young children. It presents as recurrent crops of pruritic pustules on the palms and soles. Both a bacterial infection and scabies infestation should be excluded.

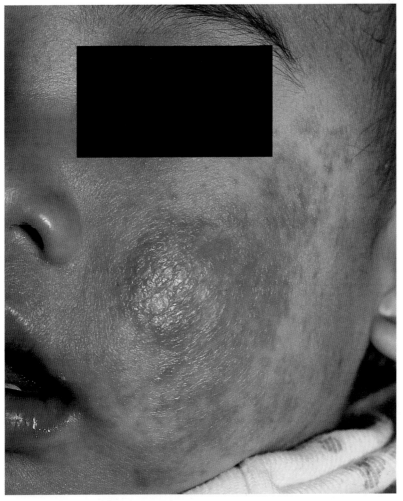

Figure 42. Atopic dermatitis, infantile, cheeks. Atopic dermatitis (AD) is a common eczematous rash affecting children with an inherited tendency toward dry skin, allergies, asthma, and hay fever. It is caused by both a defective skin barrier function and allergy to a wide variety of environmental and dietary allergens. IgE levels tend to be quite high, The patient with AD typically presents in the first few months of life with an eczematous rash. Bilaterally symmetric, red, scaly, chapped and dry, glazed cheeks are typical. An irritant dermatitis from saliva may be contributory.

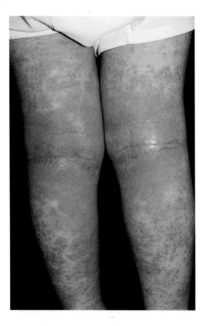

Figure 43. Atopic dermatitis, diffuse, legs. The red, scaly rash of atopic dermatitis may spread to cover much or all of the body. Often there is accentuation of the flexures, as illustrated here. The child scratches incessantly, and sleep may be significantly disrupted both for the child and for the parents.

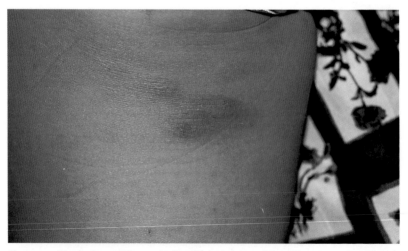

Figure 44. Atopic dermatitis, posterior, thigh. Areas of the skin commonly affected include the cheeks, neck, antecubital fossa, wrists, popliteal fossa, and the upper posterior thigh as shown here.

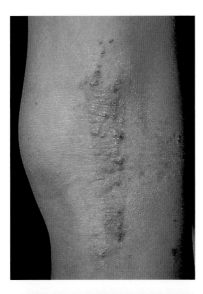

Figure 45. Atopic dermatitis, flexural with lichenification. Many of the skin changes are secondary to scratching. Linear lichenification, as shown here, and excoriations are proof that the child is scratching.

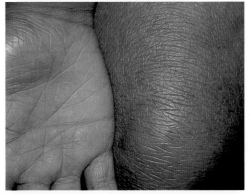

Figure 46. Hyperlinear palms and lichenification, thigh. Atopic patients often develop accentuation of the palmar creases.

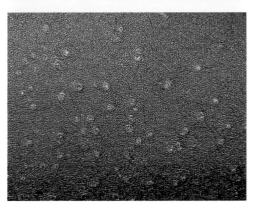

Figure 47. Follicular eczema in a dark-skinned patient. Dark-skinned patients with atopic dermatitis often show follicular accentuation. At times, only the follicles are involved, as shown here.

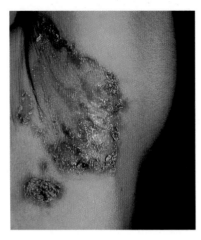

Figure 48. Atopic dermatitis, secondary infection, bacterial. Atopic skin often harbors significant numbers of *Staphylococcus aureus*. Overt infection is common and is manifested by areas of erosion, crusting or oozing, as shown here.

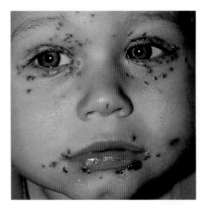

Figure 49. Eczema herpeticum, face. The patient with atopic dermatitis is predisposed to infection not only by *Staphylococcus aureus* but also by herpes simplex as shown here. Rapidly progressive, widespread crusted papules, vesicles, and erosions are characteristic of this viral infection which most commonly affects the face. (See also **Figure 371.**)

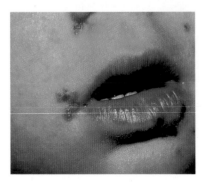

Figure 50. Eczema herpeticum, close-up. Crusted lesions in the atopic patient may represent bacterial or viral infection. At times only culture will distinguish the two. Culture of these lesions showed herpes simplex.

GENODERMATOSES: INHERITED SYNDROMES

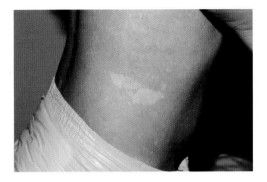

Figure 51. Tuberous sclerosis, ash leaf macule. Tuberous sclerosis is an autosomal dominant disorder characterized by skin lesions, mental retardation, and seizures. The earliest sign, the ash leaf macule, usually develops in the first year of life. It may appear as a polygonal macule, in the shape of an ash leaf or like confetti. A Wood's light aids detection of these lesions.

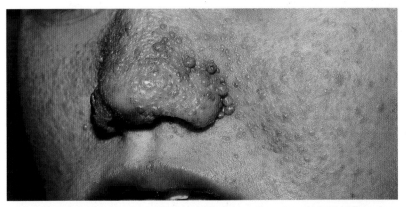

Figure 52. Tuberous sclerosis, adenoma sebaceum. Sometime during childhood or adolescence, multiple red–yellow papules begin to develop on the face of patients with tuberous sclerosis (TS) and are called adenoma sebaceum. Firm nodules and plaques on the forehead are also characteristic. Systemic manifestations of TS include cardiac rhabdomyomas, cortical or cerebral tubers, CNS tumors, pulmonary lymphangiomyomatosis, renal angiomyolipomas, renal cysts and retinal astrocytomas.

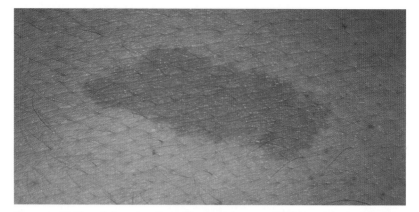

Figure 53. Café-au-lait spot. Neurofibromatosis type 1 (NF1) is an inherited disorder whose major feature is the occurrence of multiple neurofibromas, which are benign tumors of the nerve sheath. It affects an estimated one in 3000 to 4000 individuals. It is caused by mutation of the *NF1* gene which is found on chromosome 17. Two of the following seven criteria are important for diagnosis: (i) six or more café-au-lait spots (CALS), (ii) two or more neurofibromas, (iii) Lisch nodules (pigmented iris hamartomas), (iv) axillary or groin freckling, (v) optic glioma, (vi) characteristic bony deformity, and (vii) a first-degree relative with two criteria. Systemic abnormalities that may occur in neurofibromatosis include CNS tumors, pheochromocytoma, and seizures. Precocious puberty occurs in approximately 3–4% of patients and only in those with tumors of the optic chiasm. Inheritance is autosomal dominant but sporadic cases are common.

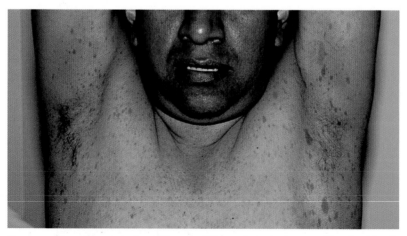

Figure 54. Neurofibromatosis, axillary freckling. Crowe's sign or axillary freckling is characteristic of neurofibromatosis.

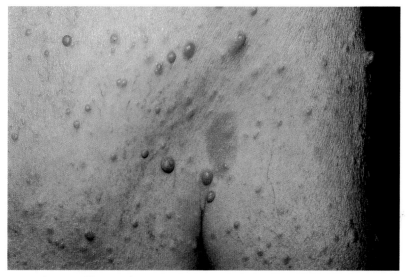

Figure 55. Neurofibromatosis, neurofibromas. Multiple to innumerable neurofibromas develop in neurofibromatosis. Neurofibromas are soft and may be 'button-holed' into the skin. A café-au-lait spot is also seen.

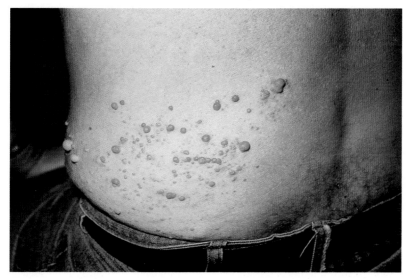

Figure 56. Neurofibromatosis, segmental. In segmental neurofibromatosis, multiple aggregated neurofibromas occur unassociated with systemic neurofibromatosis (NF). Although included here, segmental neurofibromatosis is not inherited. Instead, it is thought to represent a postzygotic somatic mutation of the primary neural crest. Clinically, one sees multiple, soft papules grouped in one area of the skin. A complete family history should be *negative* for NF, and an eye exam should *not* show Lisch nodules.

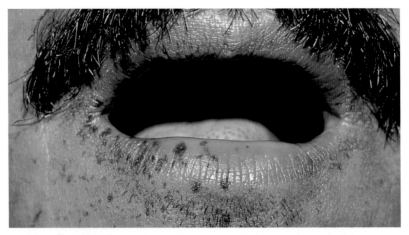

Figure 57. Peutz–Jeghers syndrome, lips.   Peutz–Jeghers syndrome (PJS) is an autosomal dominant disorder characterized by the association of mucocutaneous pigmentation and multiple gastrointestinal hamartomatous polyps and with an increased risk of developing gonadal sex tumors besides other malignancies. Pigmented macules develop in infancy or early childhood on the lips and buccal mucosa. Pigmented macules of the palm, fingers, and soles also occur. The polyps may develop from the gastroesophageal junction down to the anus, with the small bowel the most commonly affected. Their malignant potential is low. Mutation in the *STK11/LKB1* gene (a tumor-suppressor gene found on 19p13.3) is responsible for most cases of Peutz–Jeghers syndrome. (STK = serine threonine kinase.)

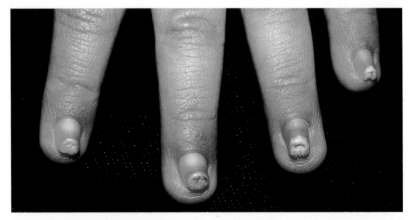

Figure 58. Pachyonychia congenita, nails.   Pachyonychia congenita is an autosomal dominant disorder in which all finger- and toenails are greatly thickened, hard and curved transversely. A mutation in one of the genes encoding keratin, *K6*, *K16*, or *K17*, is responsible for most cases, with *K6a* or *K16* mutations producing the type 1 phenotype (nail dystrophy, palmoplantar keratoderma, and oral lesions), whereas *K17* or *K6b* mutations cause the type 2 phenotype (nail dystrophy, pilosebaceous cysts following puberty, natal teeth). The nails illustrated here belong to an affected baby.

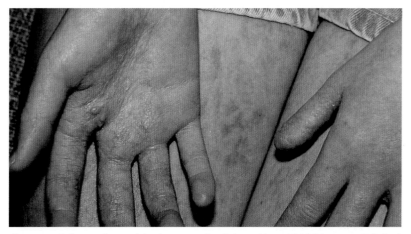

Figure 59. Goltz syndrome (also known as focal dermal hypoplasia) is a rare, X-linked dominant, multisystem disorder found almost exclusively in female patients. Congenital linear streaks of telangiectasis and atrophy, as well as soft, reddish-yellow nodules (fat herniations) are characteristic. Skeletal abnormalities such as syndactyly, polydactyly and absence of digits occur. Most patients are female.

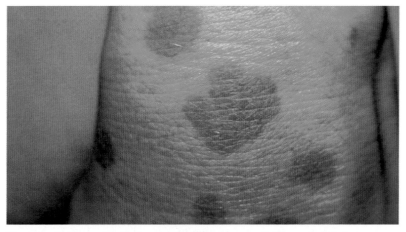

Figure 60. Epidermodysplasia verruciformis, verruca. Epidermodysplasia verruciformis is an autosomal recessive inherited disease characterized by increased susceptibility to infection by human papilloma virus (HPV), which may be found in the verruca plana lesions (pictured here), tinea versicolor lesions, and associated cutaneous malignancies (e.g. Bowen's disease or squamous cell carcinoma). HPV 5 and 8 are the most common types found in these patients. Mutations of both chromosomes 2 and 17 have been found in individual patients. (Courtesy of Steven Goldberg, MD.)

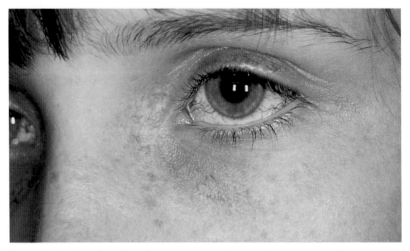

Figure 61. Ataxia telangiectasia is an autosomal recessive inherited multisystem disorder in which DNA repair mechanisms are defective, resulting in radiosensitivity, propensity to development of neoplasia, and chromosomal instability. Ocular telangiectases, as shown here, develop at 3–5 years of age. Cutaneous telangiectases develop later on the face (some visible in this patient), ears, and elsewhere. Ataxia appears when the child tries to walk. Recurrent sinopulmonary infections affect most, and bronchiectasis may develop. There is an increased risk of leukemia or lymphoma. (Courtesy of A Götz, MD.)

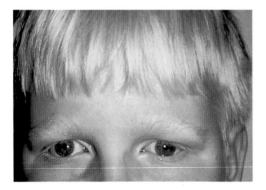

Figure 62. Albinism. Oculocutaneous albinism comprises a group of disorders with absent or deficient biosynthesis of melanin, resulting in pigmentary deficiencies of the eyes and skin. These disorders are broadly divided into tyrosine-negative and tyrosine-positive. The skin is snow white, fair or light tan, the irises may be translucent and the hair white, yellow, light brown, or red. (Courtesy of James E Rasmussen, MD.)

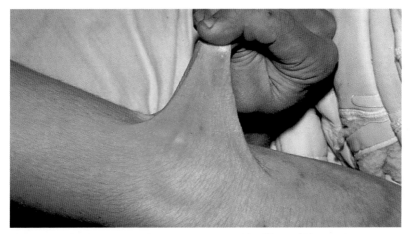

Figure 63. Ehlers–Danlos syndrome, hyperextensible skin.   Ehlers–Danlos syndrome is a group of disorders whose main abnormalities include hyperextensible and fragile skin and hyperlaxity of the joints. A specific defect in collagen production has been identified in many of the subtypes. Soft, fleshy papulonodules called molluscoid pseudotumors occur in areas subject to trauma. (Courtesy of Michael O Murphy, MD.)

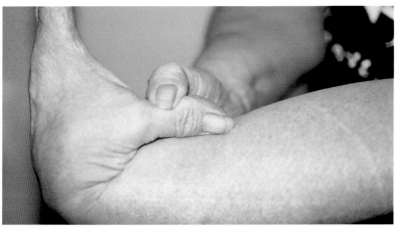

Figure 64. Ehlers–Danlos syndrome, hyperlaxity of the joints.   (Courtesy of Theodore Sebastien, MD.)

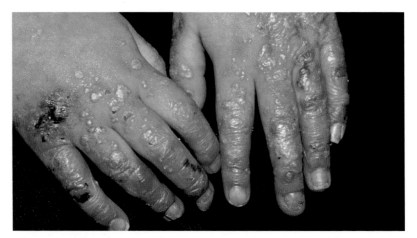

Figure 65. Epidermolysis bullosa, hands.   Epidermolysis bullosa (EB) is a family of inherited blistering skin disorders characterized by blister formation in response to mechanical trauma. Three main categories are identified based on the level of separation of the blister: EB simplex (epidermis), junctional EB (basement membrane zone), and dystrophic EB (dermis). The erosions of EB tend to heal slowly with atrophic scarring and formation of milia (small white papules). Multiple milia are seen in the healed areas of this child with EB. Many different mutations of a variety of genes have been identified.

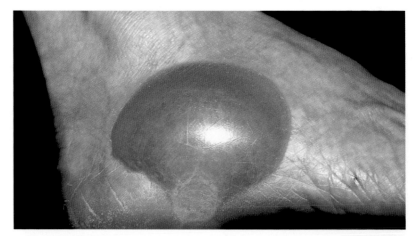

Figure 66. Epidermolysis bullosa, Weber–Cockayne.   Epidermolysis bullosa of the Weber–Cockayne subtype has a very mild presentation with blisters confined primarily to the hands and feet. There is no decrease in longevity. Blistering tends to be worse in the summer with increased sweating and friction. The patient pictured is 60 years of age.

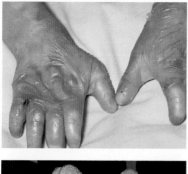

Figure 67. Epidermolysis bullosa, recessive, dystrophic (RDEB) is one of the most severe forms of EB. Repeated scarring of the digits leads to flexural contractures, digital fusion, and epidermal encasement—the so-called mitten deformity. The nails are lost early in life. In this patient, the skin is scarred, the digits short, and the nails absent. (Courtesy of Arlene Tsuchiya, MD.)

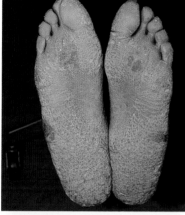

Figure 68. Keratoderma, diffuse. A variety of disorders have as part of their presentation uniform keratoderma covering the palms and soles. The pattern of hyperkeratosis may be diffuse (shown here), punctuate, or spiny. The patient shown here has the Unna Thost variant, which is inherited as an autosomal dominant condition with no other clinical findings.

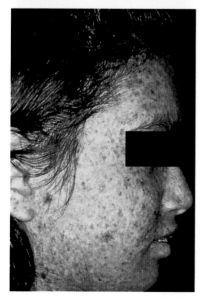

Figure 69. Xeroderma pigmentosum (XP) is a sun-sensitive and cancer-prone genetic disorder consisting of seven genetically distinct complementation groups (groups A–G). XP group D (XP-D) is a heterogeneous group. Extreme sensitivity to ultraviolet rays results from an autosomal recessive inherited defect in the enzymes involved in DNA repair. Erythema and edema after minimal sun exposure develop initially, with onset in most patients from 1–4 years of age. Later, multiple dark stellate 'freckles' and lentigos (as shown here), telangiectasia, and hypopigmented macules develop. Actinic keratoses, basal cell carcinoma, squamous cell carcinoma, and melanoma may develop and are a frequent cause of early death. (Courtesy of James Rasmussen, MD.)

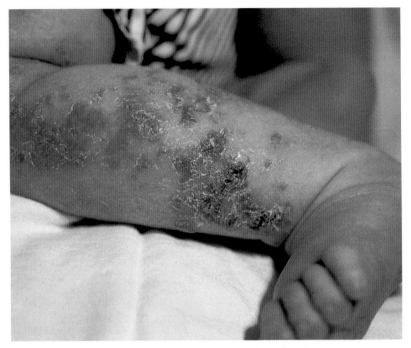

Figure 70. Incontinentia pigmenti, erosive lesions. Incontinentia pigmenti is an uncommon X-linked dominant disorder, lethal in the majority of affected males in utero, and variably expressed in females. Abnormalities of the teeth, hair, nails, eyes, and neurological system have been reported. The gene for incontinentia pigmenti has been mapped to Xq28. Female infants are affected first by erythematous, vesicular, erosive linear lesions (shown here). Soon thereafter, hyperkeratotic linear plaques (**Figure 71**) develop that finally resolve, leaving linear and whorled hyperpigmentation (see **Figure 72**). The initial vesiculobullous phase is usually present at birth or develops in the first 2 weeks of life, the verrucous second stage from the 2nd to the 6th weeks, and the third pigmentary stage is most apparent from 12 to 26 weeks. The pigmentary stage tends to fade and usually does not persist into adulthood. (Courtesy of James Steger, MD.)

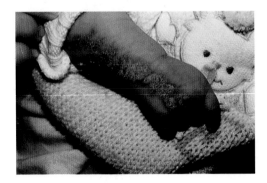

Figure 71. Incontinentia pigmenti, verrucous lesions.

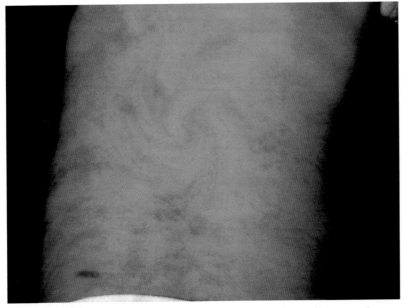

Figure 72. Incontinentia pigmenti, whorled hyperpigmentation. (Courtesy of James Steger, MD.)

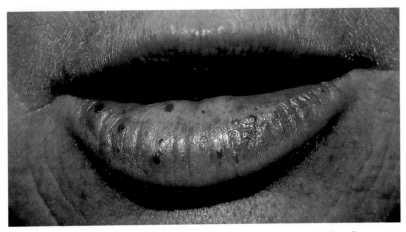

Figure 73. Hereditary hemorrhagic telangiectasia. Rendu–Osler–Weber disease, or hereditary hemorrhagic telangiectasia (HHT), is an autosomal dominant disorder with incomplete penetrance, characterized by vascular anomalies which may develop in virtually any organ. Two chromosomal sites at least have been identified: in HHT1, mutations at chromosome 9 alter the protein endoglin; and in HHT2, mutations at chromosome 12 alter the protein activine or ALK-1. The initial presentation is usually epistaxis in childhood. Later, telangiectatic mats develop on the lips (shown here), tongue, fingertips, and elsewhere. Vascular abnormalities of other organs and abscess of the CNS may occur.

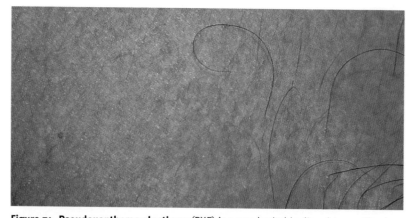

Figure 74. Pseudoxanthoma elasticum (PXE) is a rare heritable disorder resulting in the progressive calcification of elastic fibers in skin, eye, and the cardiovascular system. Mutations in the *ABCC6* (*MRP6*) gene on chromosome 16, which encodes a transmembrane transporter protein, have been shown to cause PXE. Small, yellow, reticulate papules on the sides of the neck and flexures, giving a 'plucked chicken' appearance, are characteristic. Onset is in the teenage years. Ophthalmologic and cardiac changes occur. Both mild and severe forms are seen. Inheritance is usually autosomal recessive.

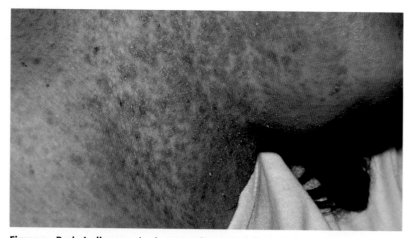

Figure 75. Darier's disease, also known as keratosis follicularis, is an autosomal dominant skin disorder characterized by abnormal keratinization and acantholysis. The causative gene has been localized to the 2-cM region of chromosome 12 and mutations have been found in the *ATP2A2* gene which encodes the sarco/endoplasmic reticulum Ca²⁺-ATPase type 2 isoform. This suggests a role for the calcium pump in a calcium signaling pathway regulating cell-to-cell adhesion and differentiation of the epidermis. The patient typically presents with scaly, waxy, greasy papules in the seborrheic area, shown here on the neck. It often worsens in the summer and may be aggravated by heat or sunlight. Onset is usually in adolescence with an autosomal dominant inheritance pattern.

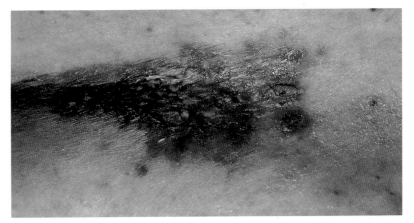

Figure 76. Hailey–Hailey disease (HHD), also known as benign familial pemphigus, is an autosomal dominant disorder with recurrent eruption of vesicles and bullae involving predominantly the neck, groin, and axillary regions. Studies have revealed that HHD is caused by mutations in *ATP2C1*, the gene encoding a novel, P-type Ca^{2+}-transport ATPase. 'Wet tissue paper' erosions or erythematous plaques are found symmetrically in the axilla and groin where the skin surfaces oppose each other. A positive family history is found in approximately 70% of cases.

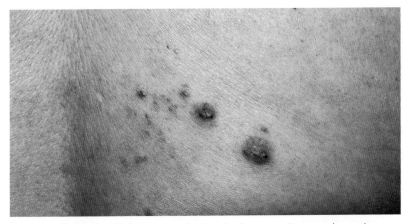

Figure 77. Blue rubber bleb nevus syndrome, also known as Bean syndrome, is a rare disorder characterized by cutaneous and gastrointestinal hemangiomas. The gastrointestinal lesions can cause intestinal bleeding and a chronic anemia. Most cases are sporadic, although some instances of an autosomal dominant inheritance pattern have been documented. The onset is usually at birth, with the progressive accumulation of lesions over time. There is no sex predilection. Most reported cases occur in Caucasians. The GI lesions may occur anywhere from the mouth to the anus, but are most common in the small intestine. Rarely, vascular tumors may develop in any of a variety of organs. The cutaneous lesions are blue or red, soft, easily compressible nodules. They may be a few millimeters to several centimeters in size. Some lesions appear as large, macular discolorations.

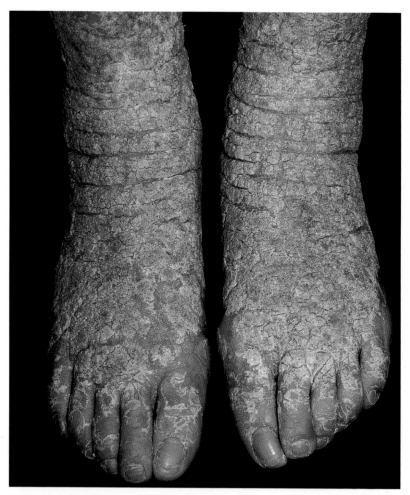

Figure 78. Epidermolytic hyperkeratosis is an autosomal dominantly inherited ichthyosis, frequently associated with mutations in *K1* or *K10* that disrupt the keratin filament cytoskeleton, leading to hyperkeratosis, blistering, and an altered barrier function. The affected infant has diffusely red, scaly skin with blister formation (which gave rise to the former name of bullous ichthyosiform erythroderma). Later, the skin becomes hyperkeratotic and verrucous diffusely as shown here in this 24-year-old woman. Significant palmoplantar keratoderma may occur, most commonly with mutations in *K1*.

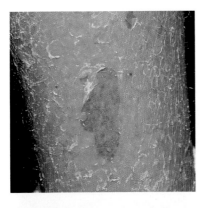

Figure 79. Epidermolytic hyperkeratosis, erosion amongst hyperkeratosis. A very helpful diagnostic sign is areas of denudation and, later, normal skin adjacent to verrucous areas.

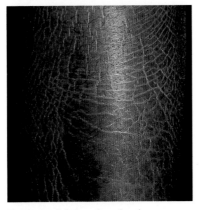

Figure 80. Ichthyosis vulgaris. Normal skin is constantly turning over, with the old cells coming to the surface and being shed. In the ichthyoses, this process is abnormal, and thickened, scaly, or hyperkeratotic skin results. The most common and the most mild of the ichthyoses is ichthyosis vulgaris. This autosomal dominantly inherited disease is most prominent on the legs and worsens in the winter. An important histological feature is an absence of the granular layer.

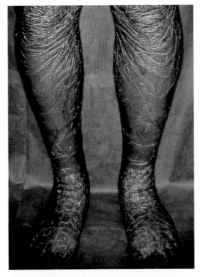

Figure 81. Lamellar ichthyosis is a congenital autosomal recessive ichthyosis which often presents as a collodion baby at birth. Many patients have been found to have a mutation in the gene (*TGM1*) encoding the transglutaminase 1 enzyme, which is responsible for assembly of the cornified envelope (CE). After the newborn period, the skin becomes ichthyotic with large plate-like scales and variable erythroderma. Ectropion and palmar/plantar keratoderma are frequently present. (Courtesy of Department of Dermatology, University of California, San Diego.)

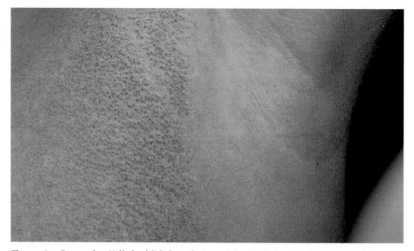

Figure 82. Recessive X-linked ichthyosis is an inherited disease due to steroid sulfatase deficiency (STS). Most patients have large deletions of the *STS* gene and flanking sequences. The scales are large, dark, and thick in this condition. The flexures are typically spared, as illustrated here. Corneal opacities may be found. Cryptorchidism and testicular cancer unassociated with cryptorchidism may occur. Only males are affected, although carrier females may exhibit mild features as well as failure to go into labor spontaneously.

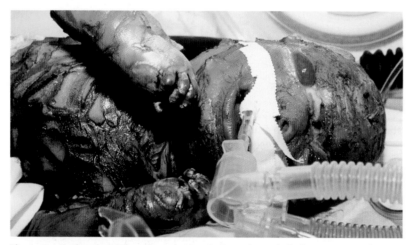

Figure 83. Harlequin ichthyosis, or harlequin fetus, is a relatively rare, severe form of congenital ichthyosis. The infant is usually premature and of low birthweight. Ectropion and eclabium are common. The ears, nose, fingers, and toes may be hypoplastic or rudimentary. The limbs may have limited mobility. Inheritance seems to be autosomal recessive. At birth, the skin is covered with hard, keratotic plates which some have likened to the crust of an apple pie. These patients almost always die in early life. (Courtesy of Angelito Arias, MD)

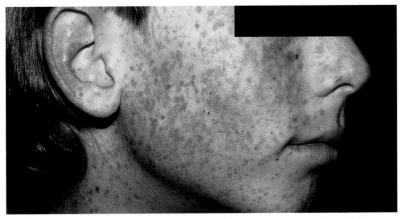

Figure 84. Freckles, or ephilides, are not normal. They are a sign of photodamage and represent an attempt by the skin to protect its DNA from excessive sunlight. The tendency toward freckling is inherited but the freckles themselves are not. Parents of freckled children should be educated on these key facts and the importance of sun protection. Light tan or brown macules scattered on the face or nose of a light-skinned, red-haired patient are characteristic.

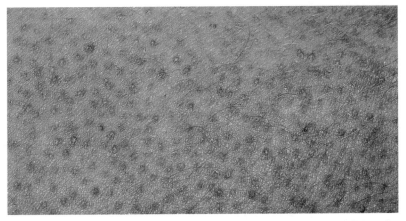

Figure 85. Keratosis pilaris, arms. Keratosis pilaris is a very common condition of children and young adults in which the hair follicles become hyperkeratotic and variably inflamed. Some reports have shown an association with high body mass index, leg skin dryness, and an atopic diathesis. The patient presents with multiple, tiny (1 mm), follicular hyperkeratotic papules, with or without erythema, on the upper, outer arms. The anterior thighs, buttocks, and cheeks may also be affected, and a diffuse truncal eruption may rarely occur.

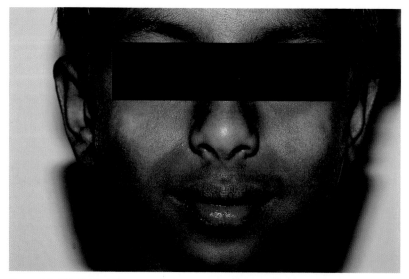

Figure 86. Pityriasis alba seems to be a variant of post-inflammatory hypopigmentation. The initial event is a patch of eczema, which may or may not be noticed. The child then presents with multiple, hypopigmented, ill-defined areas on the face and/or arms. Often there is a history of atopic dermatitis.

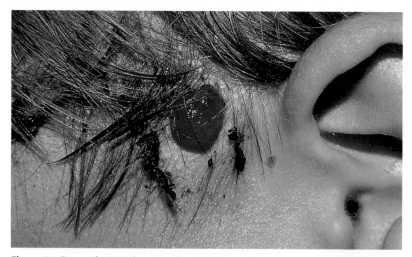

Figure 87. Pyogenic granuloma is a benign inflammatory tumor demonstrating obvious overactivity of angiogenesis. It occurs most commonly in children and pregnant women. Trauma is a common precipitating factor, but is not required. The sudden appearance of a vascular papule that bleeds easily on the finger, palm, sole, head, or neck is characteristic.

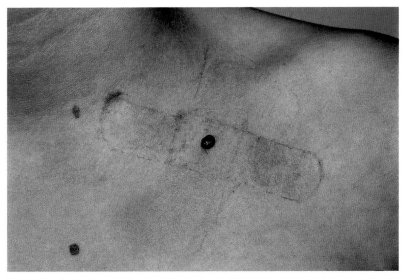

Figure 88. Pyogenic granuloma. The surface of the pyogenic granuloma is so fragile and the underlying tissue so full of blood vessels that any trauma leads to significant bleeding. Often the parent or patient applies layer upon layer of bandages to control the bleeding, giving rise to the 'bandage sign'. See also **Figure 87.**

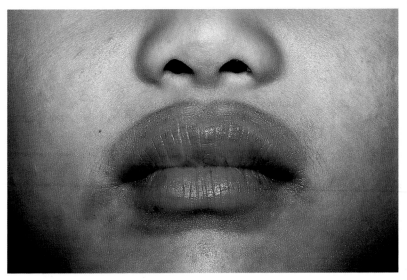

Figure 89. Liplicking represents an irritant contact dermatitis from the constant wetting and irritation by the saliva. Red, scaly, crusted, eczematous changes of the skin encircling the mouth in a child are characteristic. Only skin accessible to the tongue is affected.

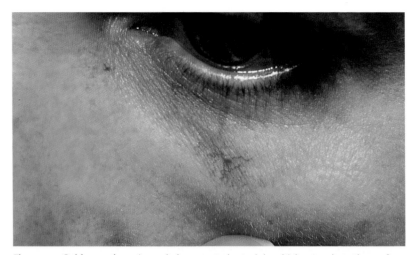

Figure 90. Spider angioma is made by a central arteriole which extends to the surface of the skin and then dissipates radially through an arcade of smaller draining vessels. Compressing the central point blanches the arcade. It is very common in children, in pregnancy, and with liver disease. The area just below the eye on the upper cheek is a very characteristic site in children, as shown here.

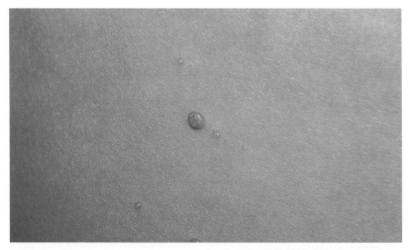

Figure 91. Molluscum contagiosum virus (MCV) is a member of the poxvirus family and causes benign skin tumors in children and immunocompromised individuals. Children 2–6 years of age may present with 2–50 pink-to-flesh-colored lesions scattered all over the body. These papules may have a smooth surface with small pinpoint areas of white studded on them, as shown here, or have a central dell (**Figure 92**), which can be brought out nicely during cryotherapy. Affected children often have a history of spending much time in the swimming pool. Molluscum may also affect patients with atopic dermatitis, adults as an STD (**Figure 350**), or patients infected with HIV (**Figures 287** and **288**).

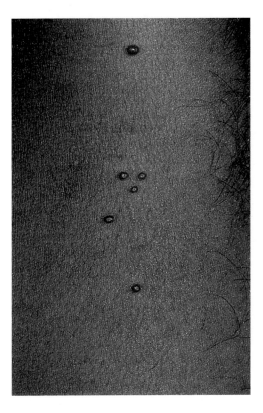

Figure 92. Molluscum contagiosum. Note the central dell on these small papules.

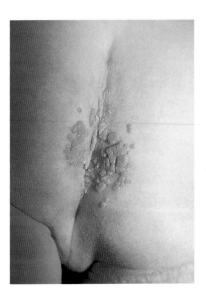

Figure 93. Condyloma, perianal.
The presence of perianal condyloma in a child 3 years or older should suggest the possibility of sexual abuse. Younger children are more likely to have received the virus from the mother during pregnancy and/or delivery. Alternative modes of inoculation include transfer from the patient's own or a parent's hand warts. (Courtesy of Michael O Murphy, MD.)

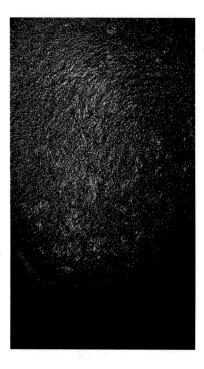

Figures 94–97. Tinea capitis (dermatophyte infection of the scalp and hair) is common in children and may present clinically in various ways, including: diffuse scale resembling seborrheic dermatitis (**Figure 94**, left); a circumscribed area of alopecia with thick crust (**Figure 95**, below); a boggy mass of tissue (kerion, **Figure 96**, top right); multiple hairs broken off at the level of the scalp (black dot ringworm, **Figure 97**, bottom right); yellow cup-shaped crusts (scutula) each pierced by a hair (also known as favus); and scattered, patchy areas of alopecia with slight scale. Note the regional lymphadenopathy in **Figure 96** that results from the tremendous inflammatory response. Wood's light fluorescence is positive in some patients. Prepubescent children are usually affected. In the USA, crowded living conditions and urban areas are risk factors. A high percentage of siblings, parents, and grandparents of the index patients are asymptomatic carriers. Most cases in the USA are caused by *Trichophyton tonsurans*.

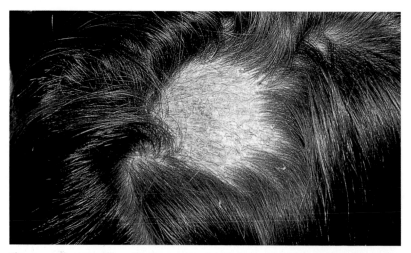

Figure 95. Tinea capitis. The fungus invades the hair, causing breakage and alopecia. The immune response is mild and thus the erythema, swelling and drainage of classic kerion (**Figure 96**) is not seen.

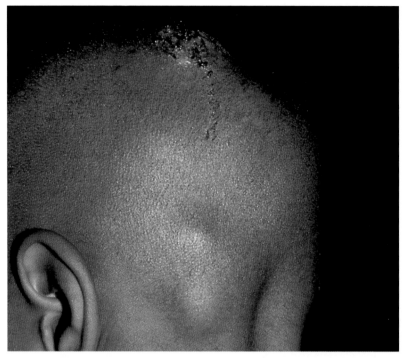

Figure 96. Kerion. When the immune response to the fungal infection is brisk, significant inflammation, swelling and tenderness develop. The term kerion is then used. The kerion is present at the top of the child's head and an enlarged lymph node is visible near the posterior neck.

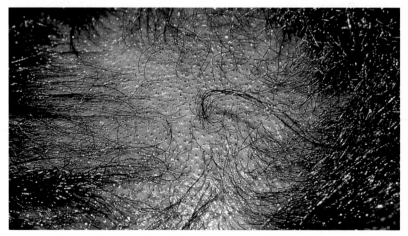

Figure 97. Black dot ringworm. If the hair breaks off at the level of the scalp, multiple black dots are seen.

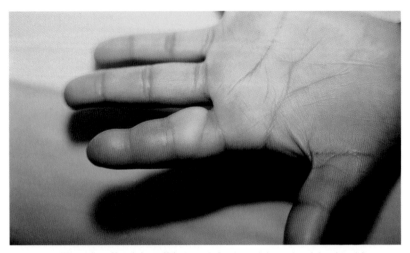

Figure 98. Blistering distal dactylitis is an infection of the pulp of the distal finger by either *Staphylococcus aureus*, group A beta-hemolytic *Streptococcus* species, or both. The patient is usually a child. Clinically, the distal volar fat pad has become one large pus-filled blister. One or more digits may be affected. (Courtesy of Arline Tsuchiya, MD.)

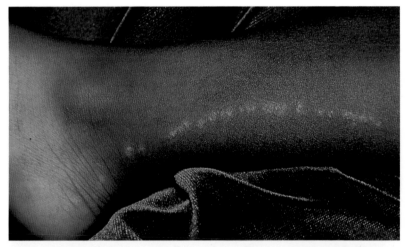

Figure 99. Lichen striatus is a benign linear inflammatory condition of unknown cause that typically affects children. The patient presents with linear papules or red, scaly lesions that follow Blaschko's lines (see **Figure 28**). In a series of 18 patients with lichen striatus, the mean age of onset was 3 years, mean duration 9.5 months, and hypochromic sequelae occurred in 50%. If the proximal nail fold is involved, nail dystrophy may occur.

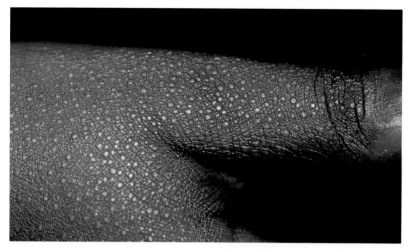

Figure 100. Lichen nitidus is an uncommon, benign papular eruption of unknown etiology. Innumerable, tiny (1 mm) papules are characteristic. Many sites may be affected. Köbnerization (lesions appearing on skin that is injured) may occur.

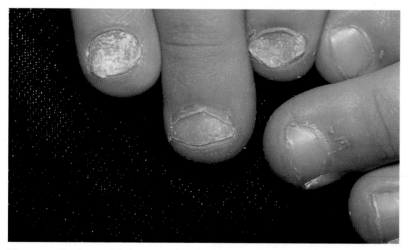

Figure 101. Trachyonychia is a term that describes a nail whose surface is diffusely rough and irregular. It may result from any inflammatory condition affecting the nail matrix, e.g. alopecia areata, psoriasis, or lichen planus, but idiopathic cases are common. Just a few or all nails may be affected. When all the nails are involved, the term 20-nail dystrophy may be used.

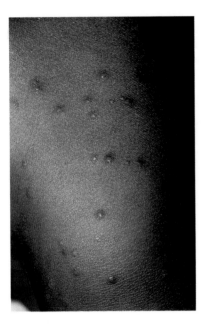

Figure 102. Papular urticaria is a common childhood disorder manifested by chronic or recurrent papules caused by a hypersensitivity reaction to the bites of mosquitoes, fleas, bedbugs, or other insects. A child will present with multiple, scattered, pruritic papules. The larger the child, the more the lesions are localized to the lower leg in the case of flea bites. Vesicles and bullae may occur. Scratching causes erosions and ulcerations. Pyoderma is common. Lesions occur in crops. (See also **Figure 410.**)

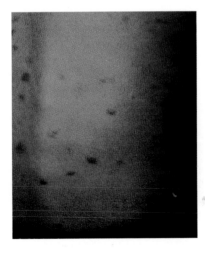

Figure 103. Urticaria pigmentosa. Mastocytosis is an abnormal proliferation of mast cells in the skin. It may occur as a solitary congenital lesion (see **Figure 18**), as multiple papules (**Figures 104** and **105**) or as hyperpigmented lesions that urticate upon stroking (urticaria pigmentosa) as shown here and in **Figure 516**. In urticaria pigmentosa, the patient presents with multiple, brown macules or papules scattered on the body. Patients may have a few to several thousand. The trunk is the most common site, followed by the extremities. Gastrointestinal or systemic histamine effects include diarrhea, stomach pain, flushing or lightheadedness. Onset in childhood is most common.

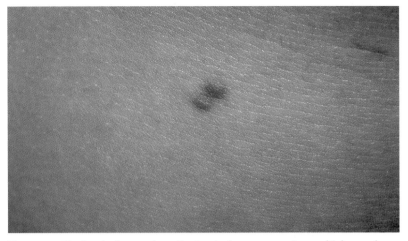

Figure 104. Mastocytosis, papule. Mastocytosis may present as multiple papules, in this case in a child.

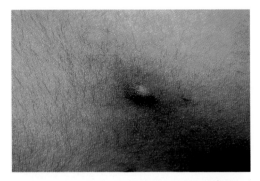

Figure 105. Mastocytosis, Darier's sign. Stroking a papule causes urtication, also known as Darier's sign. (See also **Figures 18** and **687**.)

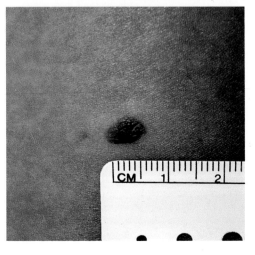

Figure 106. Spitz nevus is a benign melanocytic neoplasm of children and young adults that can be exceedingly difficult to distinguish histologically from melanoma. Clinically, it appears as a smooth, firm, red-to-brown papulonodule on the cheek of a child, but any age or body site may be affected. Some are highly vascular and mimic a hemangioma or a pyogenic granuloma.

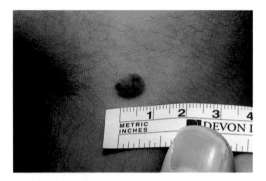

Figure 107. Spitz nevus.
This lesion is heavily
pigmented.

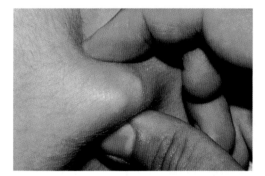

Figure 108. Pilomatricoma
(also known as the
calcifying epithelioma of
Malherbe) is an uncommon
skin tumor, believed to arise
from the hair matrix, that
occurs predominantly in
young people. A hard,
irregular, dermal or
subcutaneous tumor in a
child, often on the head or
neck, is characteristic.
It may be multiple and
familial or rarely associated
with myotonic dystrophy.
When the skin is stretched
over the skin, as shown
here, multiple nodularities
may be seen—the so-called
tent sign. Pilomatricomas
may also occur in adults.

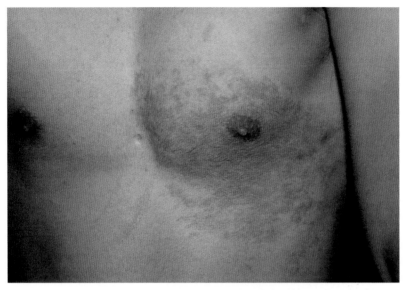

Figure 109. Becker's nevus. An acquired, unilateral, pigmented patch with irregular borders on the trunk of an adolescent is characteristic of a Becker's nevus. Hypertrichosis may develop later (**Figure 110**), and familial cases have occurred. Breast hypoplasia has occurred in lesions overlying a woman's breast.

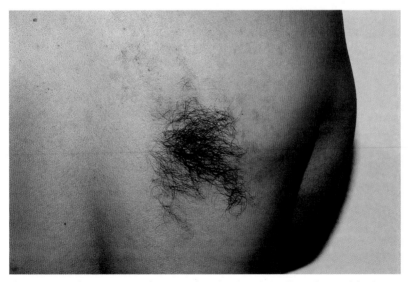

Figure 110. Becker's nevus. This nevus has developed significant hypertrichosis.

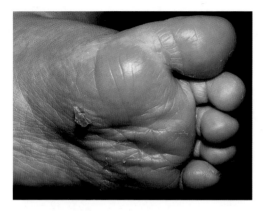

Figure 111. Juvenile plantar dermatosis is an uncommon dermatosis of the soles of young children. Atopy, friction, and alternation of the skin between wet and dry states have all been associated. Clinically, one sees shiny, cracked, erythematous areas most prominent over the toes and ball of the foot. *Tinea pedis* and shoe dermatitis should be excluded.

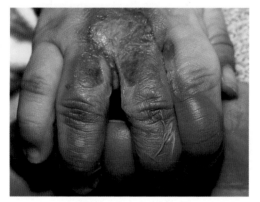

Figure 112. Child abuse. The possibility of child abuse should be considered when the child presents with acute skin changes which are asymmetric or have unusual shapes suggesting an external cause. Scalding burns, as here, or unusual bruising are typical.

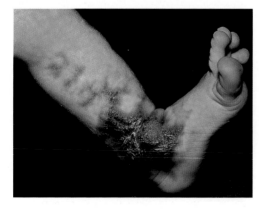

Figure 113. Cutis marmorata telangiectasia congenita is a congenital abnormality in which a localized or generalized reticulated, vascular, blue-violet network is seen clinically. In a small percentage of patients, associated anomalies occur, including body asymmetry, other vascular abnormalities, neurological anomalies (e.g. hydrocephalis, psychomotor retardation, seizures), and ocular anomalies (e.g. glaucoma).

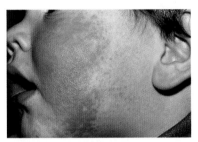
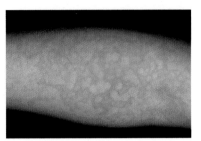

Figures 114 and 115. Erythema infectiosum.   In this infection by Parvovirus B19, a child will develop prominent erythema of the cheeks ('slapped cheeks', **Figure 114**, left) followed by a lace-like erythema on the extremities (**Figure 115**, right) and buttocks. A sore throat, cough, headache, nausea, and fever may accompany the rash. It is also known as fifth disease. Infection by Parvovirus B19 in adults may cause polyarthropathy, aplastic crisis, and hydrops fetalis.

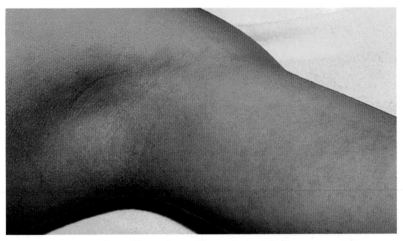

Figure 116. Asymmetric periflexural exanthem.   A scarlatiniform or eczematous eruption unilaterally on the lateral trunk and/or axilla of a child is characteristic of asymmetric periflexural exanthem. The age of onset is typically 1–3 years of age, with girls affected more commonly than boys. It may also begin in the inguinal folds, and the regional lymph nodes may be moderately enlarged. A mild fever may be present. Later, it may spread, e.g. to the other side of the thorax, the elbows, knees, and thighs, creating a symmetric distribution.

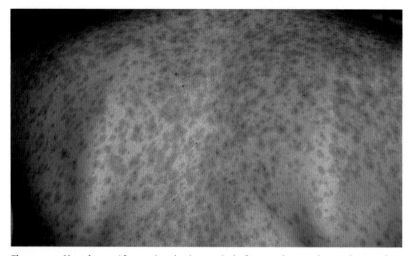

Figure 117. Measles. After an incubation period of 10–12 days and a prodrome of fever, malaise, coryza, conjunctivitis, and cough, the patient with measles will develop a maculopapular rash starting on the face and progressing to involve the trunk and extremities by the third day. Punctate whitish spots like salt grains on a red base on the buccal mucosa (Koplick's spots) are classic, developing in the prodromal period and disappearing by the height of the exanthem. Measles is caused by an RNA parmyxovirus.

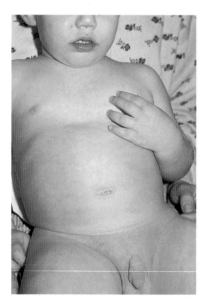

Figure 118. Kawasaki disease is an acute systemic vasculitis that has become the most common form of acquired heart disease in young children in developing countries. Increasing evidence has supported an infectious etiology; however, the debate continues as to whether the inflammatory response results from a conventional antigen or a superantigen. Five of the following six criteria are necessary for diagnosis: (i) fever for 5 days or more unresponsive to antibiotics, (ii) bilateral 'dry' conjunctival congestion, (iii) oral mucosal changes (e.g. red, crusted lips, strawberry tongue), (iv) palmar/plantar changes (e.g. erythema and edema with characteristic desquamation later), (v) polymorphous exanthem (e.g. maculopapular, scarlatiniform, erythema multiforme-like), and (vi) cervical lymphadenopathy (relatively non-tender). The patient is usually a young child. Approximately 20–25% of untreated patients develop significant cardiovascular complications including arrhythmias (acute), aneurysms, and thrombi (subacute), or scarring and ischemic heart disease (late). (Courtesy of Lon Dubey, MD.)

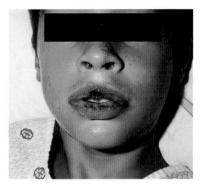

Figure 119. Kawasaki disease. Notice the swollen, inflamed crusted lips and the conjunctival infection. (Courtesy of O Dale Collins III, MD)

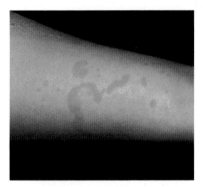

Figure 120. Urticaria in children less than 6 months of age is commonly caused by allergy to cow's milk. For children aged 6–24 months, a drug (e.g. ASA, amoxicillin) or a viral illness (e.g. hepatitis) is the most common cause. Other potential allergens in children are foods (e.g. milk, peanuts, seafood, eggs), insect bites (e.g. bees, wasps), and bacterial infection (e.g. *Streptococcus* species). (See also **Figures 679** and **682**.)

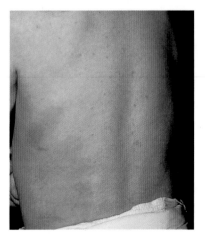

Figure 121. Roseola, also known as exanthem subitum, is a relatively benign childhood exanthem caused by human herpes virus 6, human herpes virus 7, and possibly other agents. The infant 6–18 months of age will develop a high fever but seem relatively well. Then as the fever breaks, multiple pale pink 1–5 mm macules and papules appear and last only hours to a few days.

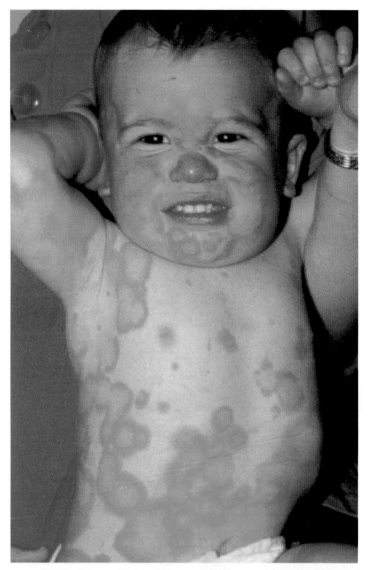

Figure 122. Serum sickness-like reaction is a specific type of drug reaction usually consisting of a unique rash, arthritis, and fever. The onset is typically 7–10 days after the causative drug was begun. It has occurred most frequently after treatment with cefaclor but may occur with other cephalosporins, penicillins, or other drugs. Clinically, one sees the acute onset in a child of inflammatory, red papulonodules that spread out into annular, urticarial plaques with dusky centers ('purple urticaria'). There are no true target lesions as with erythema multiforme, and the lesions are fixed (other than the fact that they expand) unlike urticaria. The child often has joint pains and fever. Lymphadenopathy and renal involvement usually do not occur, in contrast to a true serum sickness.

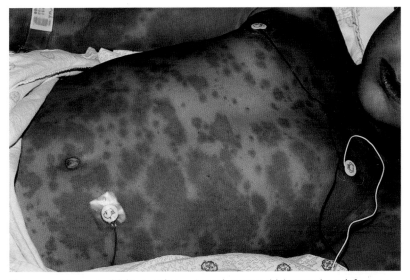

Figure 123. Hypersensitivity reaction. Some hypersensitivity reactions defy exact classification. They are typified by diffuse, symmetric, urticarial lesions that persist more than 24 hours—thus excluding urticaria. They lack purpura or necrosis that might signal a vasculitis. Many clinicians would use the term erythema multiforme, but others would object, pointing out that the lesions are not true target lesions (concentric rings of red—see **Figure 412**). Fever, malaise, and other constitutional symptoms may be present. A new drug or recent infection are the usual suspects.

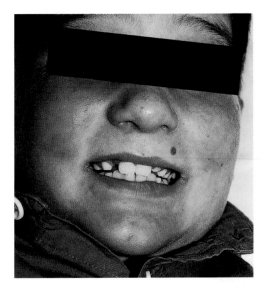

Figure 124. Juvenile dermatomyositis is a rare, chronic, multisystemic inflammatory disorder of unknown etiology, characterized by a typical skin rash and proximal muscle weakness. The disease is marked early in its course by the presence of a vasculopathy or vasculitis (e.g. of the gastrointestinal tract or myocardium), and later by the development of calcinosis. Unlike in adults, the coexistence of cancer is rare. An erythematous rash of the face and extremities is typical. Periungual erythema, Gottron's papules, and photosensitivity may occur. (See also **Figures 224** and **225**.)

Figures 125. Scarlet fever (scarlatina) is a rash caused by a toxin-producing group A beta-hemolytic *Streptococcus* species. The tonsil or pharynx is the usual site of infection, but surgical wounds or other foci are possible sites. A child typically 4–8 years of age will develop a high fever, sore throat, headache, and vomiting. The exanthem follows within 1–2 days and appears as many small papules on diffuse erythema, as shown here. The skin may feel rough like sandpaper. Linear petechiae in the axilla and groin—Pastia's lines— are classic, as is circumoral pallor. Desquamation, worse on the hands and feet, begins 7–10 days later. The tongue may be initially white and later red (strawberry tongue).

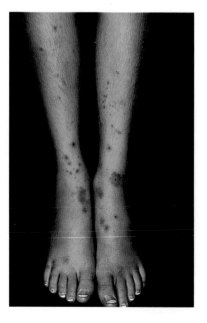

Figure 126. Henoch–Schönlein purpura is a form of systemic vasculitis characterized by vascular wall deposits, predominantly of IgA, and typically involving small vessels in the skin, gut, and glomeruli. It is associated with purpura, colic, hematuria, and arthralgia or arthritis. Viral or bacterial infections, food, or drugs are thought to be triggering events. IgA deposits may be seen on direct immunofluorescence, although this test may not be worth doing, especially in a child. Clinically, one sees a child, 3–10 years of age, who develops palpable purpura on the legs and buttocks, along with abdominal pain, vomiting, diarrhea, melena, hematuria, and arthralgias. Significant knee and ankle swelling may occur. At times, edematous, urticarial, necrotic, or hemangioma-like lesions may occur. (See also **Figure 712.**) Note the symmetric, purpuric lesions on the legs of this child.

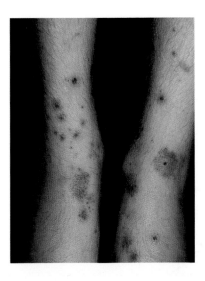

Figure 127. Henoch–Schönlein purpura. Close-up of purpuric lesions.

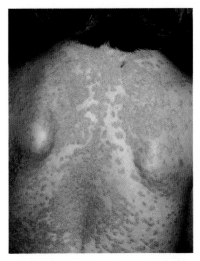

Figures 128 (left) **and 129** (below). **Guttate psoriasis** is the most common type of psoriasis in children and is characterized by the sudden development of disseminated 0.5–2.0 cm, red, scaly papules or small plaques. An upper respiratory tract infection is a very common precipitant. The disease may remit spontaneously or proceed to chronic plaque-type psoriasis. Both children pictured here are 5 years of age. Note the residual post-inflammatory hypopigmentation in **Figure 129**. (See also **Figure 539**.)

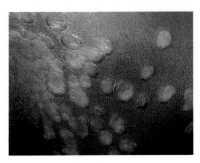

Figure 129. Psoriasis. Chronic plaques of psoriasis are shown. There is minimal scale. Where lesions have resolved, post-inflammatory hypopigmentation remains.

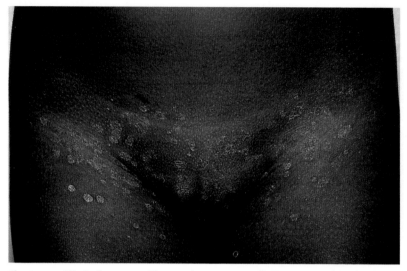

Figure 130. Pityriasis rosea. The papulosquamous papules and plaques of pityriasis rosea commonly affect children and young adults. The groin is a preferred site as illustrated in this 5-year-old girl. (See also **Figures 552–556**.)

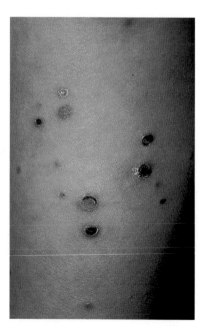

Figure 131. PLEVA is an acronym for pityriasis lichenoides et varioliformis acuta. The characteristic lesion is initially a red papule that develops a hemorrhagic and necrotic center. Lesions of all stages occur and are illustrated on this child's leg. Fever and constitutional symptoms may accompany the outbreak.

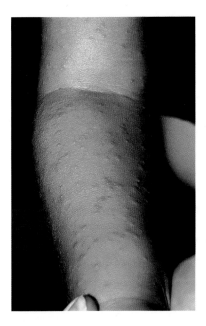

Figure 132. Gianotti–Crosti syndrome.
Papular acrodermatitis of childhood, also known as Gianotti–Crosti syndrome, is a self-limiting disorder with acute-onset generalized lymphadenopathy and a symmetric erythematous papular and papulovesicular eruption of the face, neck, buttocks, and extremities, usually occurring in young children. This rash usually results from an underlying viral infection, e.g. Epstein–Barr, varicella, coxsackie, cytomegalovirus, or hepatitis.

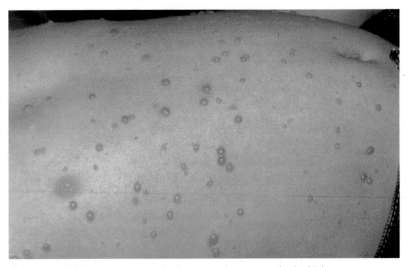

Figure 133. Chickenpox. The varicella zoster virus causes both chickenpox (varicella) and shingles (herpes zoster). The child develops crops of several to hundreds of vesicles, each like a drop of water on an erythematous base on the trunk, face, extremities, and oral mucosa. Headache, malaise and fever may accompany the rash. Systemic involvement is more common in adults and may consist of pneumonia, hepatitis, glomerulonephritis, encephalitis, and arthritis.

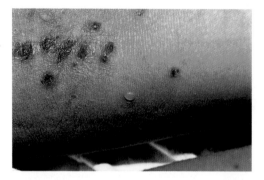

Figure 134. Bullous impetigo. Cutaneous infection by *Staphylococcus aureus* causes inflammation and a honey-colored crust (see **Figure 48**). If an epidermolytic toxin is produced by the bacteria, vesicles and bullae may form, as shown here.

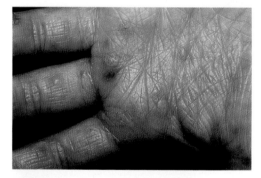

Figure 135. Hand, foot, and mouth disease. Hand, foot, and mouth disease is a self-limiting, childhood, bullous eruption caused by a viral infection (usually by coxsackie A-16). Typically, one sees 3–8 mm gray–white oval vesicles on the hands, feet, and buttocks. Aphthae-like erosions occur in the mouth. A low grade fever, malaise, and lymphadenopathy may occur. Epidemics are common.

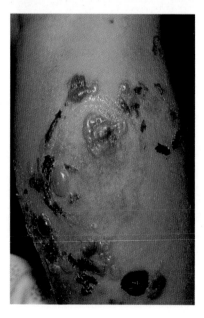

Figure 136. Chronic bullous disease of childhood is an autoimmune blistering disease occurring in prepubertal children and characterized by a linear deposition of IgA along the basement membrane zone. Clinically, one sees large bullae, often in rosettes or in clusters of 'jewels'. The perioral and genital area are often affected. Unlike dermatitis herpetiformis, a gluten-sensitive enteropathy is not associated.

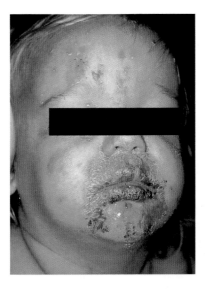

Figure 137. Staphylococcal scalded skin syndrome is caused by a localized infection of *Staphylococcus aureus* that secretes an exfoliating toxin. This toxin acts as a serine protease which cleaves desmoglein 1, causing skin at sites distant from the infection to become erythematous and tender followed by superficial desquamation. The face may be heavily involved (giving the impression that someone hit the patient in the face with an 'impetigo pie'). The skin may desquamate in large sheets. Toxic epidermal necrolysis should be excluded (see **Figure 243**). (Courtesy of Eliot Mostow, MD.)

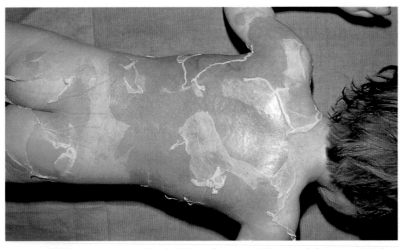

Figure 138. Staphylococcal scalded skin syndrome. Widespread desquamation is seen. (Courtesy of James Rasmussen, MD.)

For related diseases, see also herpes zoster in a child (**Figure 377**).

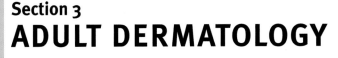

Section 3
ADULT DERMATOLOGY

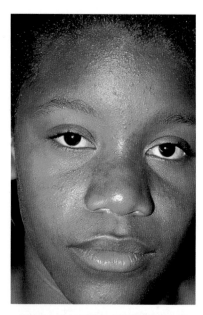

Figure 139. Acne vulgaris, mild/comedonal. Classic teenage acne begins around age 10–14 years as open and closed comedones (blackheads and whiteheads, respectively) of the central face. Increased sebum production, proliferation of *Propionibacterium acnes*, and abnormal keratinization of the follicular epithelium are the principal contributory factors.

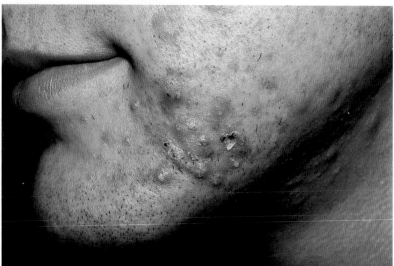

Figure 140. Acne vulgaris, moderate, inflammatory. As the acne progresses, lesions become more numerous, larger, and more inflammatory.

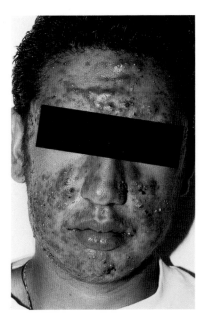

Figure 141. Acne vulgaris, severe.
In severe acne, large nodulocystic lesions abound. Scarring will certainly occur. The severity of acne for males peaks in the 15–17 age range and usually remits by 20 years of age. Unfortunately for females, acne may last well into the twenties, thirties and forties.

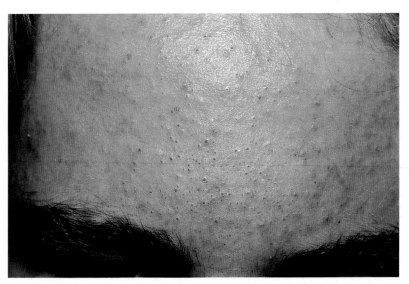

Figure 142. Acne vulgaris, open comedones.   The opening of the follicle is clogged by lipid and cellular debris. The black color of open comedones represents melanin (not dirt!).

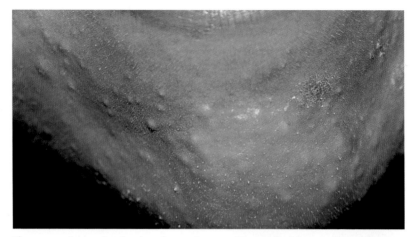

Figure 143. Acne vulgaris, closed comedones. The small white papules on this woman's chin represent closed comedones. They are often not very apparent unless the skin is stretched, as shown here.

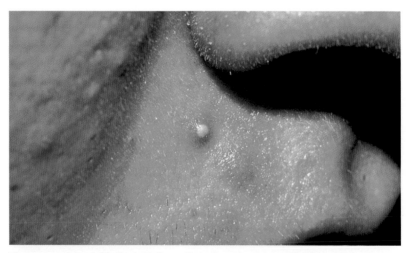

Figure 144. Acne vulgaris, pustular. Mounting pressure and inflammation can rupture the follicle, extruding its inflammatory contents into the dermis. The body's immune system mounts an intense response to wall off the insult. This process converts a non-inflammatory comedone to an inflammatory papule, pustule, or nodule.

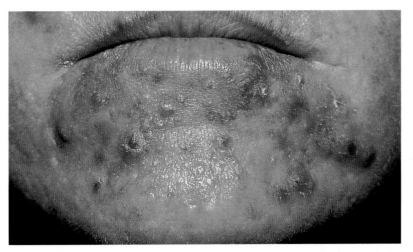

Figure 145. Acne vulgaris, papulopustular, scarring. Deep, inflammatory papules and nodules can cause significant scarring. Young adult women, as the one pictured here, are commonly affected along the jaw line and chin.

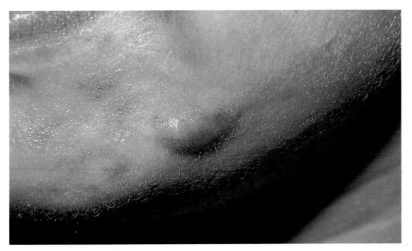

Figure 146. Acne vulgaris, nodulocystic. Ruptured follicular contents and an associated intense inflammatory response can cause extensive tissue destruction. An acne 'cyst' may result. The 'cystic' acne lesion is not a true cyst, as it lacks an epithelial wall. The bulging abscess may be fluctuant, but incision and drainage causes additional scarring.

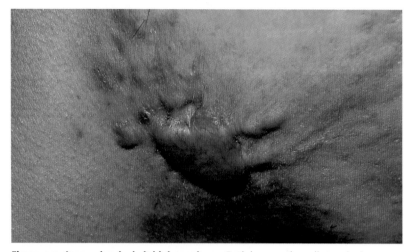

Figure 147. Acne vulgaris, keloidal scarring. Both large and small acne lesions can produce significant scarring. Scars may be atrophic, 'ice pick', hypertrophic, or keloidal as shown here.

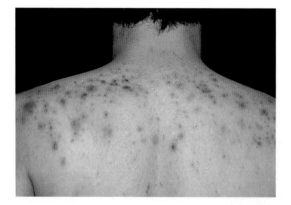

Figure 148. Acne vulgaris, back. The upper back is a common site for acne, especially in young adult men. Erythematous papules and nodules predominate, and comedones are inconspicuous. Mechanical factors may play an etiologic role. This variant tends to respond less well to conventional therapy.

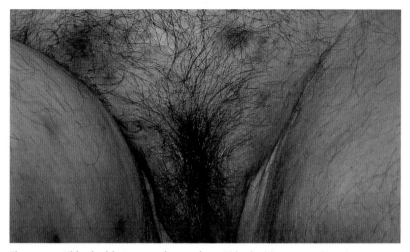

Figure 149. Hidradenitis suppurativa, groin. Hidradenitis suppurativa, acne conglobata, and dissecting cellulitis of the scalp constitute the follicular occlusion triad. Some add the pilonidal sinus to make a tetrad. These conditions may occur alone or in combination. This woman suffered from repeated bouts of inflammatory nodules of the groin and infra-mammary area.

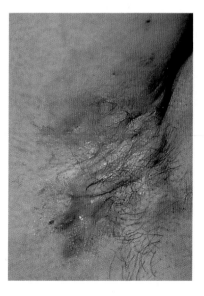

Figure 150. Hidradenitis suppurativa, axilla. Despite its name and the fact that hidradenitis suppurativa affects areas inhabited by apocrine glands, it appears to be caused by poral occlusion of the pilosebaceous unit with inflammation of the apocrine glands occurring secondarily. Patients will present with inflammatory nodules and sterile abscesses of the axilla, the groin, infra-mammary area, and/or the perianal area. Later, with chronic inflammation, sinus tracts, fistulas, and hypertrophic scarring develop, as shown here. Smoking, obesity, heat, sweat, and friction all trigger or exacerbate the condition.

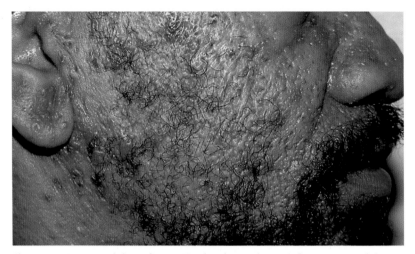

Figure 151. Acne conglobata, face.   Fistulated comedones, inflammatory nodules with pus, scarring, and sinus tracts of the back, buttocks, face, and chest occur in acne conglobata. This disease most commonly affects young males. The dividing line between severe acne and acne conglobata is not always clear.

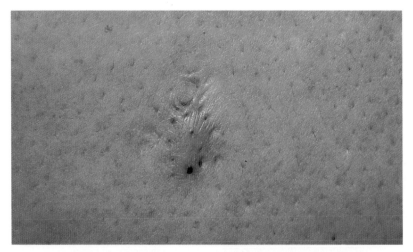

Figure 152. Fistulated comedone.   The larger comedone with multiple openings is characteristic of acne conglobata and occurs in greatest numbers on the back. It actually forms by the merging of multiple sebaceous follicles via an inflammatory process, and represents a scar. The only effective treatment of this lesion is to unroof the cavity.

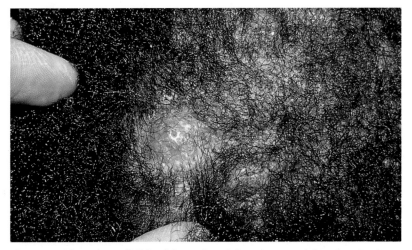

Figure 153. Dissecting cellulitis of the scalp.   Inflammatory nodules, sinus tracts, chronic drainage, and sclerosing alopecia occur in this disease, also known as perifolliculitis capitis abscedens et suffodiens. Tufts of hair may emanate from a single opening. A chronic bacterial infection, usually by *Staphylococcus aureus*, is typical and in many cases may be the primary cause.

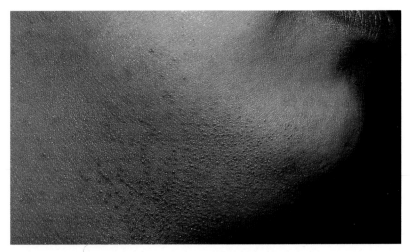

Figure 154. Hirsutism refers to the presence of excessive body hair in a woman. The presence of acne and hirsutism together should suggest the possibility of an underlying endocrinologic abnormality. Menstrual abnormalities and androgenic alopecia may also be found. This woman shaves in order to control her condition.

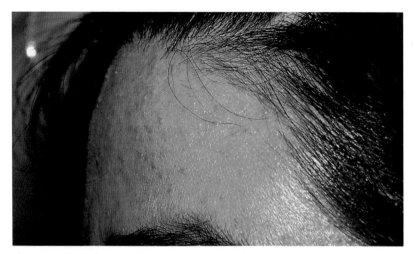

Figure 155. Pomade acne refers to acne that is precipitated by the application of cosmetics to the skin. When the acne is concentrated on the forehead and/or temples, a comedogenic hair substance is often found. Mousses, gels, and conditioners are common offenders.

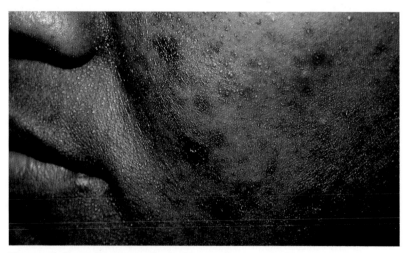

Figure 156. Post-inflammatory hyperpigmentation. Dark-skinned patients frequently develop hyperpigmented macules at the sites of previous acne lesions. Resolution usually takes months.

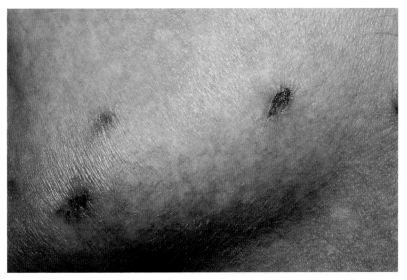

Figure 157. Excoriations in acne.   Some acne patients are unable to keep their hands away from their face. Multiple excoriations are the result. The physician can learn quickly to recognize these patients by the large red spots their fingernails leave, as shown here. Patients with no underlying acne but who still scratch their face must be excluded.

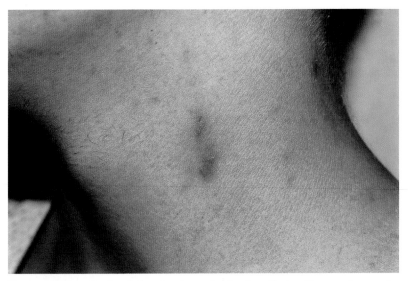

Figure 158. Sinus tract.   A sinus tract may develop in patients with acne. It presents as a linear inflammatory lesion that fails to clear with standard therapy. Treatment is usually surgical. Note the slight indentation at the top of this linear red lesion which marks the opening.

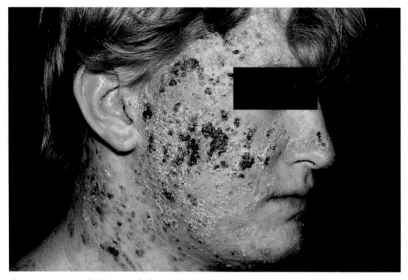

Figure 159. Acne fulminans (AF) is a rare, explosive variant of acne that typically affects Caucasian boys, 13–16 years of age. They usually have a history of mild acne but present with the acute onset of inflammatory nodules on the chest and back that may break down leaving crusted ulcerations. Virtually all patients complain of fever, arthralgias, and myalgias. Bone pain is common, and osseous defects may be present. AF may be precipitated by isotretinoin therapy (as shown here), testosterone therapy, or it may develop without any obvious trigger factors. Pyogenic granuloma lesions may form in the crusts.

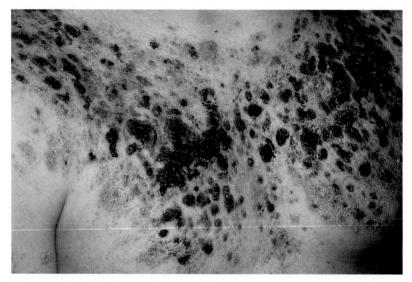

Figure 160. Acne fulminans.   Close-up of the chest, showing pyogenic, granuloma-like lesions.

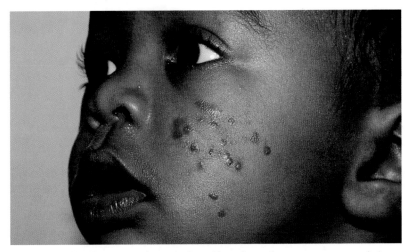

Figure 161. Infantile acne. The typical manifestations of acne may occur rarely in a child, usually male, with onset from 3 to 6 months. The face is primarily affected with comedones, small papules, pustules, and even deep-seated papules and nodules. Congenital adrenal hyperplasia or a virilizing tumor should be excluded.

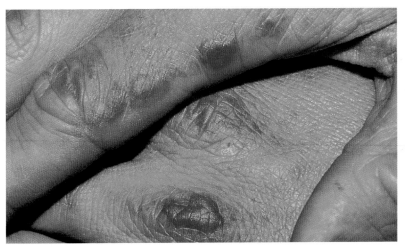

Figure 162. Photodermatitis, doxycycline. Doxycycline is known for its ability to cause significant sun sensitivity. The nose and back of the hands are most commonly affected by confluent erythema and, when severe, blistering as shown here.

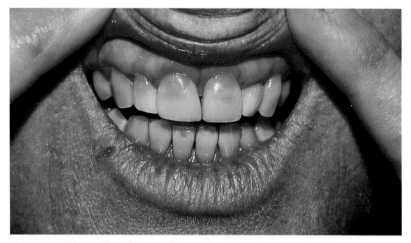

Figure 163. Minocycline pigmentation, teeth.   Chronic minocycline therapy can cause various parts of the body to turn blue, including the teeth, nails, scars, sclera, and skin. Facial acne scars as well as scars from other trauma may be affected. Patients on higher doses, e.g. 100 mg twice a day, are at greatest risk. This patient had been receiving minocycline for 15 years.

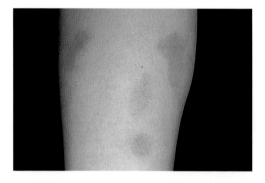

Figure 164. Minocycline pigmentation, legs.   These patches are usually thought by the patient to be bruises, and in fact they probably started out that way. However, once the iron from the blood is outside of the vascular system, it chelates with minocycline. Over time, the lesion becomes too blue and persistent to still be thought of as a bruise.

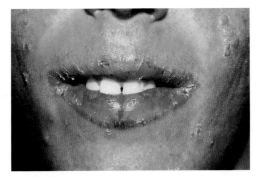

Figure 165. Isotretinoin cheilitis. Isotretinoin is a powerful retinoid used to treat acne. It is highly efficacious, but has many side effects, the most significant being damage to an unborn fetus if the woman becomes pregnant. Less serious but more common side effects include dry skin, cheilitis (shown here), muscle aches, low back ache, and dry eyes. By greatly decreasing sebum production by the skin, oral isotretinoin also increases the risk of cutaneous infection by *Staphylococcus aureus*.

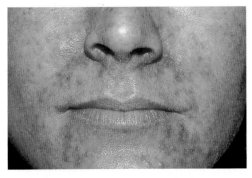

Figure 166. Periorifacial dermatitis is a papular eruption of the face affecting young women. It has many features of rosacea both clinically and histologically. Clinical features are tiny erythematous papules, pustules and a small amount of scale about the mouth. Confluent erythema of the nasolabial fold is a classic sign, and a narrow zone above the lips is typically spared. Comedones are absent. The use of a potent topical steroid may trigger or contribute to the eruption. The classic story is of a patient who can reduce the rash significantly with the use of a potent topical steroid, but the moment she stops, the rash flares again badly.

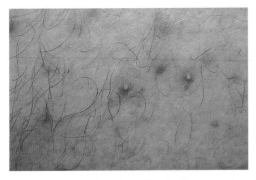

Figure 167. Steroid acne usually begins several weeks after the administration of systemic corticosteroids. Follicular papules and pustules develop primarily on the trunk. The lesions tend to be monomorphous, and comedones are usually absent. It has been proposed that many cases of steroid acne represent a pityrosporum folliculitis, as this organism may be cultured in significant numbers in the follicle, and the condition often responds well to oral antifungal agents, e.g. itraconazole.

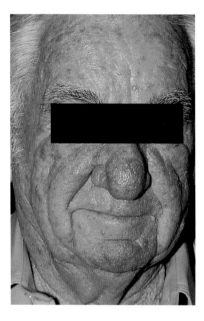

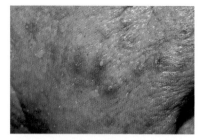

Figures 168 (left) **and 169** (above).
Rosacea is a common facial acneiform disorder affecting middle-aged and older adults, particularly the fair-skinned. The cause is not known, but response to antibiotics (e.g. tetracycline) is so rapid that an infectious agent seems likely. Erythematous papules and occasional pustules are scattered symmetrically on the face, particularly on the nose and cheeks. Comedones are absent. At times, the nose may be so involved as to turn completely red. Telangiectases may accumulate over time, and ocular involvement may occur. Many patients have a significant flush or blush of the cheeks that may be precipitated by hot liquids. Ocular rosacea is characterized by red and dry eyes.

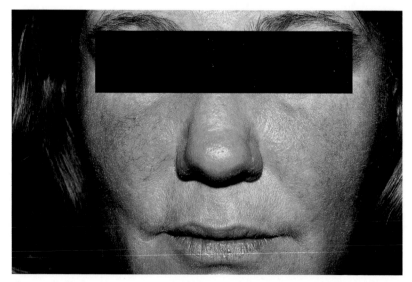

Figure 170. Not rosacea.   Facial telangiectases without papules or pustules do not constitute rosacea. Standard medical treatment of rosacea has no effect. Occasionally, this presentation is confused with the malar rash of lupus.

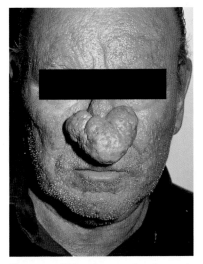

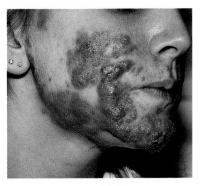

Figure 172. Rosacea fulminans.
The acute onset of large, deep, inflammatory nodules and abscesses on the face of a young adult woman is characteristic of rosacea fulminans, formerly called pyoderma faciale. The chin, cheeks, and forehead are preferentially affected. In contrast to acne fulminans, constitutional symptoms, comedones, and typical acne lesions on the chest and back are absent.

Figure 171. Rhinophyma. In advanced stages of rosacea, significant and disfiguring dermal hypertrophy may occur. The most common of these swellings or 'phymas' is rhinophyma, as pictured here. (Courtesy of Michael O Murphy, MD.)

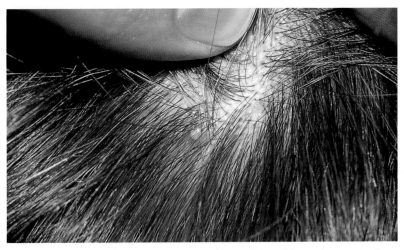

Figure 173. Acne necrotica is a common pustular condition of the scalp seen most commonly in middle-aged men. The cause is unknown, although some cases may be variants of rosacea. Both crusted papules and pustules develop. The patient often picks the lesion so quickly that the clinician only gets to see the crusted aftermath. Facial lesions along the hairline also occur.

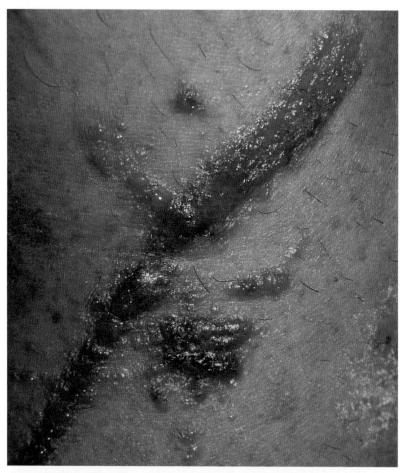

Figure 174. Rhus dermatitis. Allergic contact dermatitis (ACD) refers to inflammation of the skin caused by a T-cell-mediated allergic response to some allergen that has come in contact with the skin. The initial eruption is microvesicular and extremely pruritic. Signifiant swelling, drainage, and bulla formation may subsequently occur. Different areas of the skin erupt at different times depending in part on the severity of the allergen exposure. A classic sign of ACD is linear lesions that do not follow Blaschko's lines (see **Figure 28**) (but instead follow the pattern of exposure to the allergen). Note the linear pattern in this patient who came into contact with poison oak.

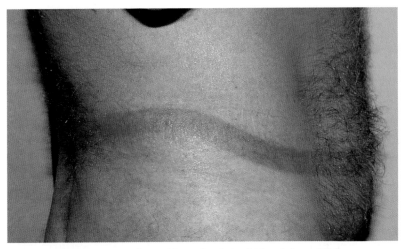

Figure 175. Allergic contact dermatitis to elastic (waist band dermatitis).
Elastic may become very allergenic when bleached. This red, pruritic eruption is
unmistakably related to elastic in the patient's underwear. The eruption did not
develop until his wife bleached the patient's underwear, a classic history. There is no
way to salvage the underwear; it must be thrown away.

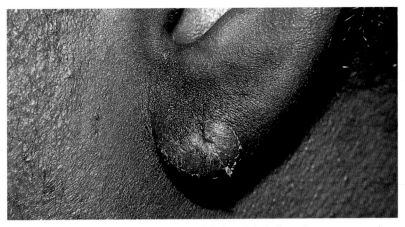

Figure 176. Allergic contact dermatitis to nickel.　Nickel allergy is very common in
women because of their long term exposure to nickel in jewelry. The ear lobes may
become pruritic, inflamed, and eczematous if earrings contain nickel. Lichenification
may result from chronic rubbing. Other areas in contact with nickel-containing metal
may react. When told they have an allergy, patients often protest, saying they have
used the item for years without trouble. But it is usually only after years of exposure
that the patient develops the allergy.

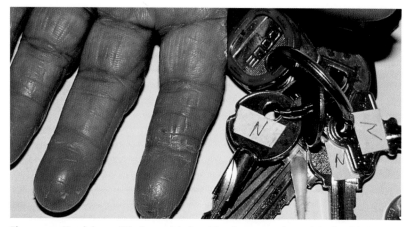

Figure 177. Hand dermatitis from nickel. Allergic contact dermatitis should always be considered in a patient presenting with an eczematous eruption. The hands are a common site for both allergic and irritant contact dermatitis because they come into contact with so many things. Patch testing in this patient showed a nickel allergy. Three of her keys tested positive to dimethylglioxime (a method to determine if an item contains nickel). Changing keys greatly improved the eruption.

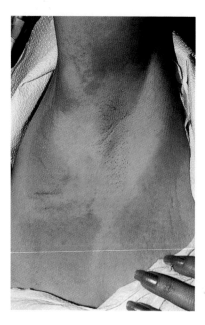

Figure 178. Clothing allergy.
New clothes are often treated with compounds to make them wrinkle free. If the clothing is not washed first, the patient may develop an allergic contact dermatitis. When the rash occurs near the axilla, it classically spares the vault as shown here. Washing the article solves the problem.

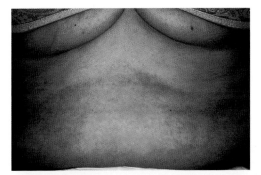

Figure 179. Dye allergy.
This woman developed an allergy to disperse blue 124 clothing dye. Note the sparing of the skin protected by the bra and breast. (Courtesy of Daniel Shaw, MD.)

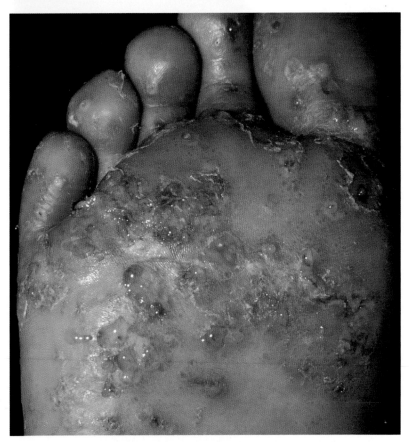

Figure 180. Shoe dermatitis mimicking pompholyx. This 10-year-old boy was treated for several years with the diagnosis of 'severe pompholyx'. It was only when patch testing was performed that an allergy to mercaptobenzathiozole was found. Rubber-free shoes cleared the feet completely! Shoe dermatitis is common in boys who sweat excessively. The moisture more easily allows the shoe allergens to come in contact with the skin.

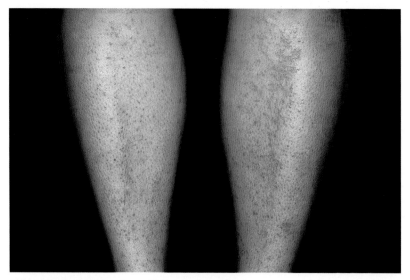

Figure 181. Body lotion dermatitis.   An increasingly common rash in women is a contact dermatitis to a body lotion. This increase arises from the growing use of body lotions containing ingredients such as fruits, berries, and herbs. Within several days, the patient will develop an intensely pruritic papular rash where she has applied the body lotion.

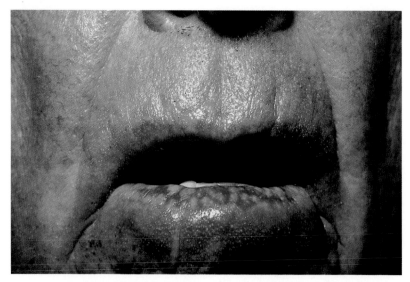

Figure 182. Cinnamic aldehyde dermatitis.   Cinnamic aldehyde is a common fragrance additive in foods and various health and beauty products. Cinnamic aldehyde in toothpaste may cause allergic contact dermatitis of the lips and perioral area. The patient will present with either a cheilitis, as shown here, or a rash simulating perioral dermatitis.

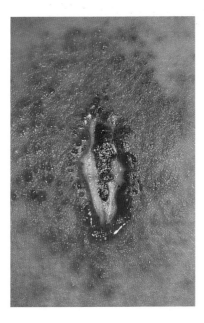

Figure 183. Bacitracin allergy.
Allergic contact dermatitis to wound care ointments and bandages may mimic a postoperative wound infection. Intense itching, a microvesicular, eczematous rash, distribution according to the pattern of contact by the bandage and/or salve, and relative lack of pus are helpful diagnostic signs. This patient developed redness, inflammation and dehiscence 10 days after a minor surgical excision. Allergic contact dermatitis to bacitracin was the cause.

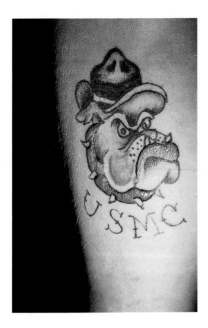

Figure 184. Tattoo allergy. Rarely, a patient will be allergic to the tattoo pigment. Reaction to the red pigment, cinnabar (mercuric sulfide), is most common. (Courtesy Michael O Murphy, MD.)

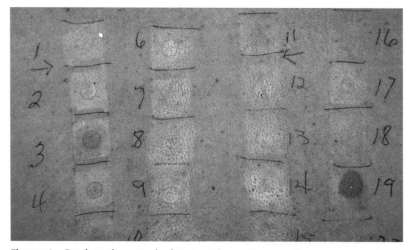

Figure 185. Patch testing, standard tray.   When cutaneous allergy is suspected, patch testing should be done. Patches containing a standard tray of allergens are applied to the back for 48 hours. In this case, allergens 3 and 19 reacted.

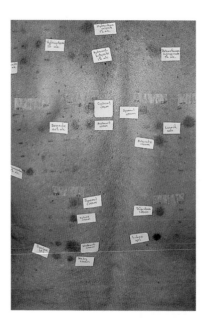

Figure 186. Patch testing, topical steroids.   Patch testing beyond the standard tray is often necessary. All of the compounds being tested here are topical steroids. This patient reacted to over 20! Extended patch testing may be done in a variety of categories, including fragrances, metals, preservatives, etc.

OCCUPATIONAL MEDICINE

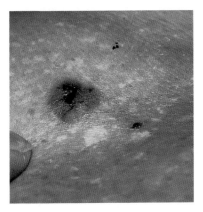

Figure 187. Non-melanoma skin cancer. Contact dermatitis and non-melanoma skin cancer are the most common occupational skin disorders in North America. Those occupations that require the most sun exposure predispose to skin cancer and include lifeguards, postal workers, and construction workers. Actinic keratoses, basal cell carcinoma (shown here), squamous cell carcinoma, and melanoma may all occur.

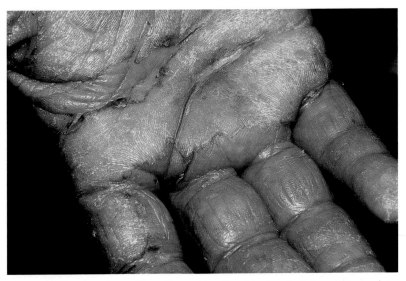

Figure 188. Paraben dermatitis. Occupationally related contact dermatitis may be either irritant or allergic. Typical findings of a work-related condition are that it worsens with work and clears or improves during vacations. Often, extensive study of the work place and examination of material data sheets is necessary to solve the clinical problem. This patient developed a severe hand dermatitis unresponsive to standard therapy. Patch testing revealed an allergy to paraben in the hand cleanser at work.

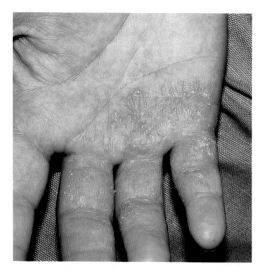

Figure 189. Rubber dermatitis. This patient underwent patch testing because his hand dermatitis would clear up on vacation and return once he resumed work. A rubber allergy was found. His job was to count and bundle money which required him to hold a rubber band around his hand in the area of the dermatitis.

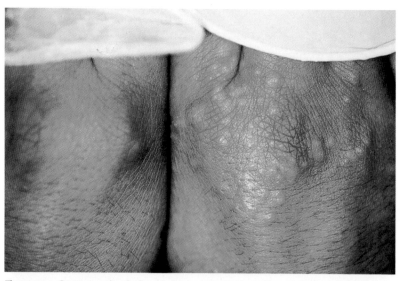

Figure 190. Contact urticaria from latex. Latex is the milky colored sap from the Brazilian rubber tree. Because of its strength and elasticity, it is used in a wide variety of medical products. Unfortunately, allergy to latex is a growing problem. Patients who are latex-allergic develop urticarial lesions from seconds to up to 45 minutes after exposure. Asthma and anaphylaxis may also occur. Food allergies commonly coexist, e.g. to avocados, bananas, kiwi, papaya, or chestnuts. Balloons, rubber balls, and condoms may be a source of latex as well. This woman developed urticaria on the right hand 5 minutes after contact with a latex glove; by contrast the vinyl glove control on the left hand is negative. (Courtesy of Daniel Shaw, MD.)

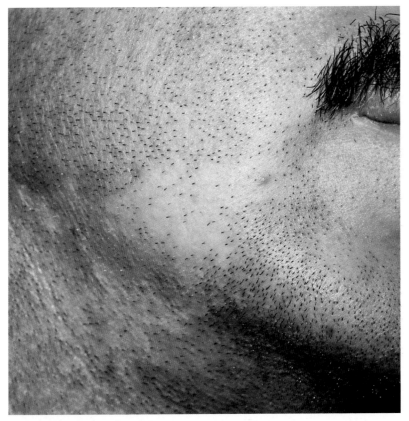

Figure 191. Chemical leukoderma.   When they come in contact with the skin, various chemicals can induce a white spot or leukoderma. Potential offenders include hydroquinones, catechols, phenols, or mercaptoamines. These are commonly found in cleansers and pesticides. The patient shown here developed facial depigmentation from a disinfectant that contained orthophenylphenol and para-tertiary amphylphenol. Other causes of chemical leukoderma include diphenylcyclopropenone (used by some to induce allergic contact dermatitis in treating, e.g., alopecia areata), and paraphenylene diamine (used in hair-coloring products). The changes of chemical leukoderma may be indistinguishable from vitiligo (see **Figures 503–506**).

BLACK DERMATOSES

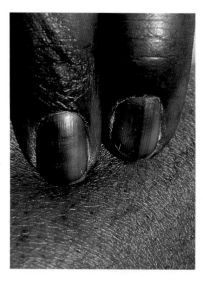

Figure 192. Longitudinal melanonychia. A longitudinal, pigmented streak of the nail commonly occurs in dark-skinned patients and is usually benign. Rarely, melanoma may occur. Benign lesions tend to be multiple, narrow bands uniformly colored, occurring in younger people, whereas malignant lesions tend to be solitary, wide, dark and/or multicolored in an older person. See also **Figures 453** and **454**.

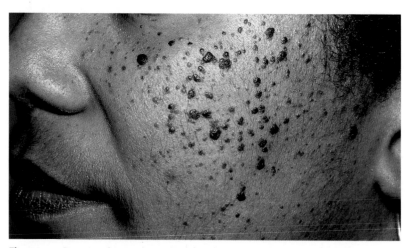

Figure 193. Dermatosis papulosa nigra (DPN) is a common papular condition of the face and neck in darker-skinned patients. Histologically, DPN appear as seborrheic keratoses. Clinical features are multiple, brown, papules, small plaques, and pedunculated lesions on the face, neck, and upper trunk.

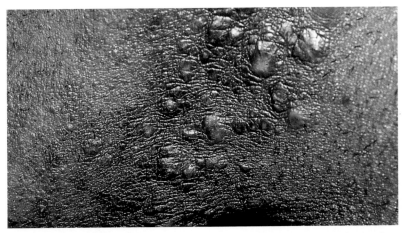

Figure 194. Pseudofolliculitis barbae. Papules and pustules in the beard area of a dark-skinned patient who tries for a close shave is characteristic. The curly whiskers curl into the skin, causing swelling and inflammation. Shaving often cuts or traumatizes these papules, adding to the problem.

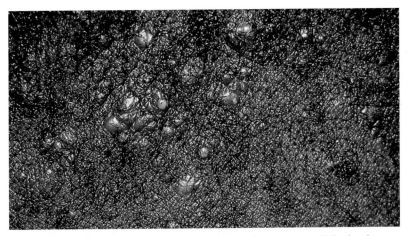

Figure 195. Acne keloidalis nuchae. A young dark-skinned man initially develops a follicular, pustular eruption on the nape of the neck. Shaving the head and wearing a collar may precipitate the condition. Keloidal formation is signaled by the development of firm, follicular papules. The coexistence of pseudofolliculitis barbae has been noted in many patients.

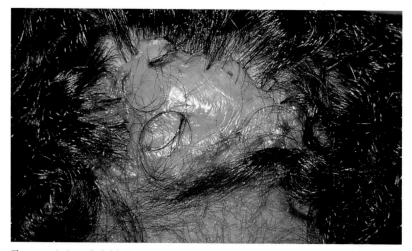

Figure 196. Acne keloidalis nuchae. Large keloids may form as well as polytrichia (tufts of hair emanating from the same opening), sinus tracts, pus, and scarring alopecia.

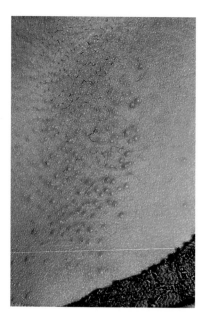

Figure 197. Fox–Fordyce disease is an uncommon, chronic, follicular-based papular dermatosis confined to apocrine gland-bearing skin. Uniformly distributed, pruritic, flesh-colored papules in the axilla, areola, groin, and perineum are characteristic. Women at puberty or later are typically affected, with men developing lesions only one-tenth as often.

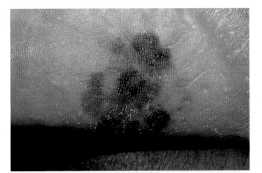

Figure 198. Acral melanoma. Melanoma in dark-skinned patients is rare, but when it does occur, the palms, soles, and nails are preferred locations. This lesion on the sole had grown slowly over several years.

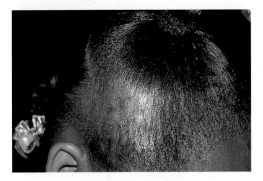

Figure 199. Traction alopecia. This term refers to loss of hair that has been subject to chronic tension. The alopecia typically starts at the edges of the section of hair involved where the traction is the greatest, e.g. at the hairline. Inflammation is usually not seen, although follicular pustules may occasionally occur. Over time, scarring occurs and the alopecia becomes permanent. Young dark-skinned girls who wear tight pony tails or braids are most commonly affected. Adults often show permanent alopecia bitemporally.

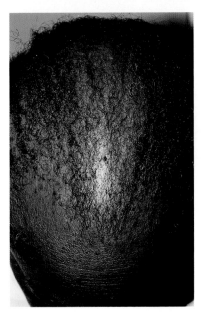

Figure 200. Follicular degeneration syndrome is a common cause of scarring alopecia in the darker-skinned woman. For years it was called hot-comb alopecia. Now it is clear that a darker-skinned woman may develop a scarring alopecia unrelated to how she cares for her hair. The scalp across the top and front is most commonly affected by hair loss and follicular dropout. Men may rarely be affected.

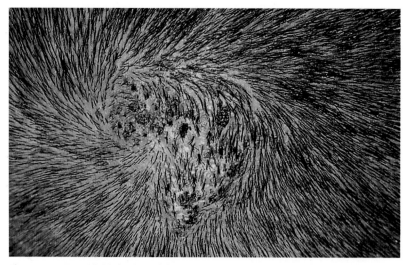

Figure 201. Bacterial infection of the scalp. The vertex of the scalp is prone to infection by *Staphylococcus aureus*, particularly in dark-skinned patients. Extensive scarring, alopecia, and tufting of hair may occur. See also **Figure 153**, dissecting cellulitis of the scalp.

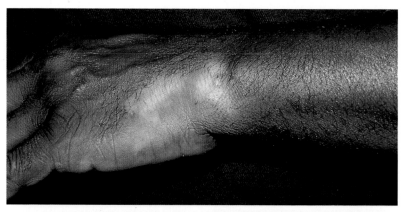

Figure 202. Steroid-induced hypopigmentation. Dark-skinned patients may develop localized hypopigmentation from either the application of a high potency topical steroid or from intralesional corticosteroid injection (as was done in this case into the wrist joint).

For related diseases, see also follicular eczema (**Figure 47**) and dermatosis papulosa nigra (**Figure 437**).

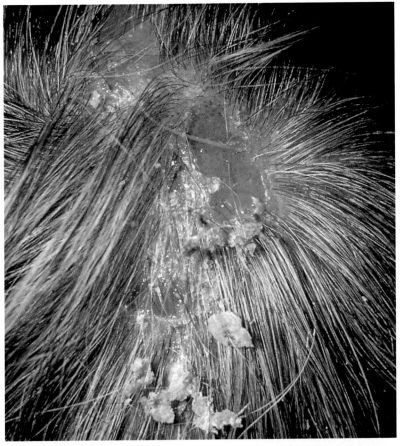

Figure 203. Pemphigus vulgaris, erosions, scalp. Pemphigus vulgaris (PV) is an autoimmune blistering disorder caused by circulating antibodies to epidermal adhesion molecules. The separation is intraepidermal, and direct immunofluorescence shows intercellular IgG and/or C3. Indirect immunofluorescence (IIF) is usually positive, and its titer may correlate with disease activity. Clinically, one sees widespread, flaccid bullae and crusted erosions in a middle-aged patient. Oral involvment is much more common in PV than in bullous pemphigoid. Untreated PV has a high mortality rate. Drug-induced PV is well recognized. Most drugs which induce or flare pemphigus are thiols (SH-containing). Some sulfur-containing drugs can undergo metabolic changes to create thiol metabolites, e.g. piroxicam, penicillins, and cephalosporins. Some drugs capable of inducing pemphigus do not have a thiol but do have an active amide group (e.g. dipyrone, enalapril). Finally, gold and penicillamine can induce PV. (Courtesy of Robert Butler, MD.)

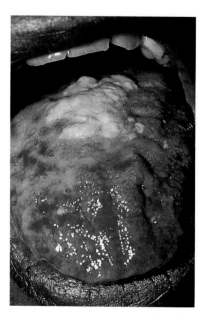

Figure 204. Pemphigus vulgaris, tongue. Oral erosions are very common in pemphigus vulgaris. Indeed, the patient may present with only oral ulcerations. Eating may be impaired.

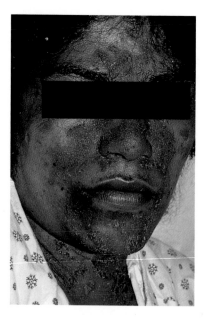

Figure 205. Pemphigus foliaceous (PF) is a superficial blistering disorder caused by antibodies primarily to the type 1 isoform of desmoglein—an important component of desmosomes (specialized domains of the plasma membrane that play a fundamental role in intercellular adhesion). The separation is in the upper epidermis, and direct immunofluorescence shows intercellular IgG and/or C3. Clinical features are erosions, bullae, and crusted plaques affecting the face, chest, and elsewhere. Some patients may have their disease exacerbated by UV-light exposure. Drug-induced PF may occur. Causative medications include fosinopril, an angiotensin-converting enzyme inhibitor (ACE inhibitor), nifedipine, and penicillamine. An endemic type also known as fogo selvagem occurs primarily in Brazil and mainly affects children and young adults.

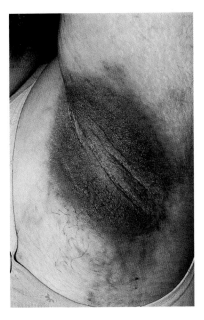

Figure 206. Pemphigus vegetans, axilla. Pemphigus vegetans is a rare variant of pemphigus which is mainly localized in the intertriginous areas (e.g. groin, axilla). Flaccid bullae and erosions which progress to vegetating, malodorous plaques are characteristic. Sulci and gyri on the dorsum of the tongue (called cerebriform tongue) have been described. Pemphigoid vegetans, which appears to be a variant of bullous pemphigoid, is clinically similar. Occasionally, drugs may be associated, e.g. enalopril or captopril.

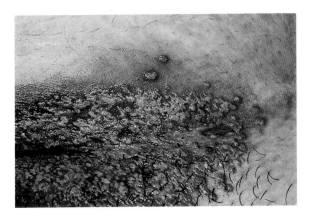

Figure 207. Pemphigus vegetans, groin. Moist, confluent vesicles and erosions in the groin are seen.

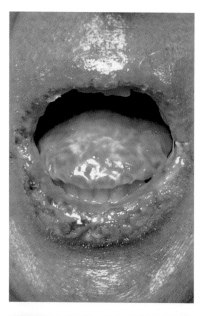

Figure 208. Paraneoplastic pemphigus, oral cavity. Paraneoplastic pemphigus is an autoimmune blistering and erosive mucocutaneous disease associated with neoplasia. Extensive erosions of the oral cavity, conjunctiva, vagina, and lips are characteristic. The mucosal erosions frequently extend beyond the vermilion border of the lips, as illustrated here. Average age of onset is 60 years. Associated neoplasms include bronchogenic squamous cell carcinoma, non-Hodgkin's lymphoma, and chronic lymphocytic leukemia among others. Mortality is high. (Courtesy of WP Daniel Su, MD, and reproduced with permission from *Journal of the American Academy of Dermatology*, 1994; 30:841–4.)

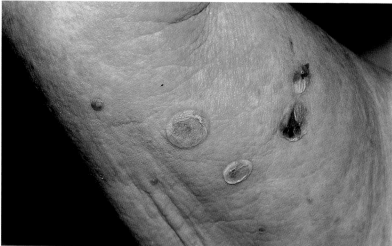

Figure 209. Bullous pemphigoid (BP) is the most common autoimmune blistering dermatosis, affecting mainly the elderly, and is associated with autoantibodies to the hemidesmosomal bullous pemphigoid antigens 180 and 230. The separation is subepidermal, and direct immunofluorescence shows IgG and/or C3 along the basement membrane zone. The patient may present initially with urticarial plaques (see **Figure 679**) which then develop thick-walled bullae (as shown here). Oral involvement is less common than in pemphigus vulgaris. Drugs, in general, do not cause BP, although a variety of reports indicate this may rarely occur (e.g. furosemide, penicillamine, captopril, etc.). Both topical and oral iodine have been reported to cause BP.

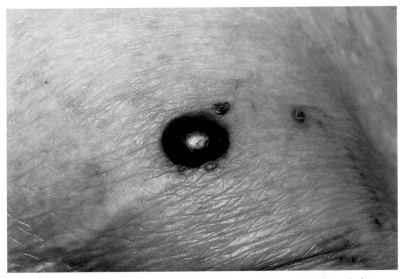

Figure 210. Bullous pemphigoid. Because the separation is subepidermal, the bullae may be large, tense, and even hemorrhagic as shown here.

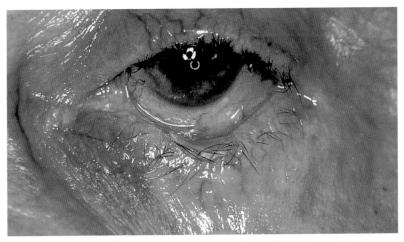

Figure 211. Cicatricial pemphigoid, eye. Cicatricial pemphigoid is an autoimmune blistering disease that predominantly involves mucous membranes with resultant scar formation. The level of separation is subepidermal, and direct immunofluorescence shows IgG and/or C3 at the basement membrane zone. IIF may be positive. The eye may be affected by a chronic conjunctivitis, burning, and excessive tearing. Later, conjunctival shrinkage, entropion, corneal opacities, and trichiasis may occur. If untreated, fibrous adhesions may attach both lids to the eye and ultimately blindness can develop. (Courtesy of Eliot Mostow, MD.)

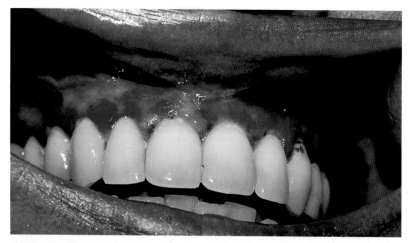

Figure 212. Cicatricial pemphigoid, gums. The oral mucosa is also commonly involved, causing oral ulceration and/or a desquamating gingivitis, as pictured here. The nasal, pharyngeal, laryngeal, esophageal, and/or anogenital regions may be affected as well.

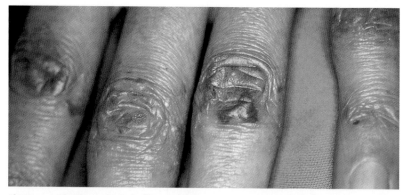

Figure 213. Epidermolysis bullosa acquisita is an autoimmune blistering disease of the skin characterized by IgG autoantibodies against type VII collagen. Clinical features are trauma-induced bullae, milia, and atrophic scars symmetric on the dorsa of the hands, feet, and elbows. Some patients may develop mutilating acral involvement with scarring and syndactyly. The patient's serum characteristically reacts to the dermal side of salt-split skin. The disease may be confused clinically with bullous pemphigoid or porphyria cutanea tarda (PCT). Urinary porphyrins help exclude PCT, and immunofluorescence with split skin helps exclude bullous pemphigoid. (Courtesy of Eliot Mostow, MD.)

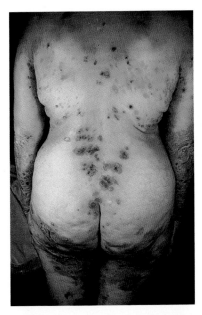

Figure 214. Dermatitis herpetiformis is an autoimmune disease mediated by granular IgA deposits in the papillary dermis. The separation is subepidermal, and direct immunofluorescence is usually positive for IgA in the dermal papillae. Gluten, the presumed causative antigen, is a protein found in most cereals, except rice and corn. A gluten-sensitive enteropathy is present, and most patients have villous atrophy, although most do not have diarrhea. Clinically, one sees a chronic, intensely pruritic vesicular rash that affects the knees, sacrum, back, posterior axillary folds, and the elbows symmetrically. Vesicles may not be found as the patient may scratch them away. (Courtesy of James Steger, MD.)

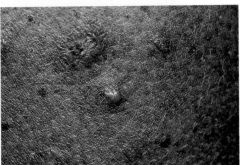

Figure 215. Dermatitis herpetiformis. When bullae do form, they are usually very small (as shown here) and last only a short time. Soon, because of the intense itch, the patient will scratch them away.

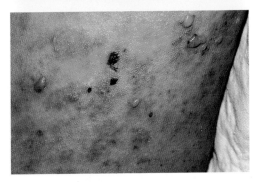

Figure 216. Bullous lupus erythematosus Vesicles and/or bullae may rarely occur in a patient with systemic lupus erythematosus. The bullae are subepidermal and have clinical similarities to those of bullous pemphigoid or dermatitis herpetiformis. Circulating IgG which reacts to type VII collagen is found. Direct immunofluorescence shows IgG at the basement membrane zone. Children may rarely be affected.

CONNECTIVE TISSUE DISORDERS

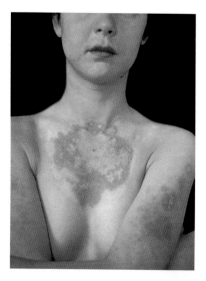

Figure 217. Systemic lupus erythematosus, butterfly rash.
SLE is a multi-system autoimmune connective tissue disease characterized by the presence of antinuclear antibodies. Clinically, one sees bilateral erythema of the cheeks and malar eminences (butterfly rash) or a more extensive photodistributed rash. Other findings include discoid rash, oral ulcers, photosensitivity, renal disease, neurological disease, arthritis, serositis, hematologic disorders, or immunologic disorders. (Courtesy of James Steger, MD.)

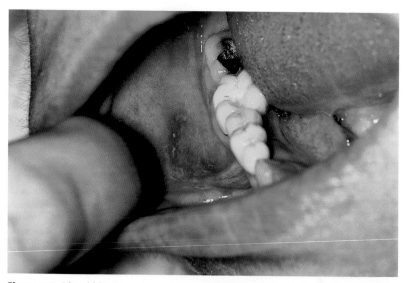

Figure 218. Discoid lupus erythematosus, oral ulceration. Oral ulcerations may occur in both systemic and discoid lupus erythematosus.

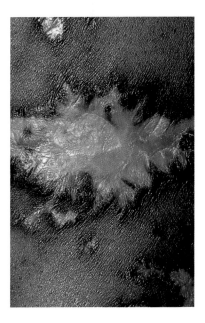

Figure 219. Discoid lupus erythematosus (DLE, also known as chronic cutaneous lupus erythematosus) is a variant of lupus in which the disease affects mainly the sun-exposed areas of the skin. SLE should be excluded. Clinically, one sees erythematous and scaly or hyperkeratotic lesions occurring in photoexposed areas. The scale may fill the follicular orifices and, if confluent, may be peeled back and the undersurface found to resemble the undersurface of a carpet (so-called carpet-tack sign). The border is often hyperpigmented, as illustrated here, and significant scarring may occur. Significant atrophy may develop over time. A recent report found that a high percentage of patients with DLE are smokers.

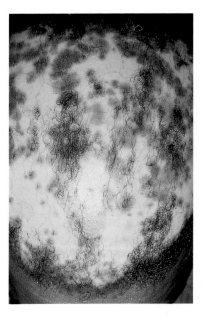

Figure 220. Discoid lupus erythematosus, alopecia. Significant scarring alopecia may occur in DLE. (Courtesy of Michael O Murphy, MD.)

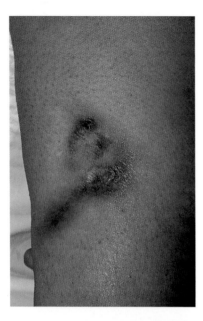

Figure 221. Lupus profundus.
Lupus erythematosus profundus is an unusual variant of cutaneous lupus erythematosus that is characterized by chronic, recurrent inflammation of the underlying fat, leading to lipoatrophy and significant depression. The upper, outer arm is a characteristic site. The overlying skin may be relatively unaffected or show changes typical of DLE.

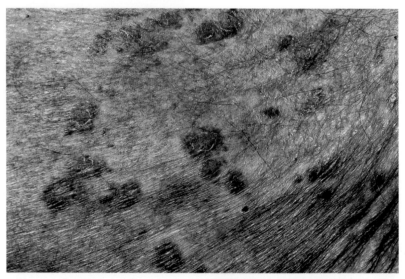

Figure 222. Subacute cutaneous lupus erythematosus, psoriasiform lesions.
Subacute cutaneous lupus erythematosus (SCLE) is a distinct variant of lupus erythematosus characterized by photosensitivity and anti-SS-A/Ro antibidies. Severe renal or CNS disease usually is not associated. One should exclude drug-induced SCLE (e.g. from hydrochlorothiazide). Arthritis is common (40–75%). The majority of patients are women. Clinically, one may see a papulosquamous rash in the photo-exposed areas (as shown here) or annular lesions (**Figure 223**).

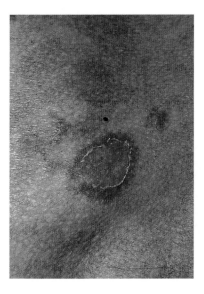

Figure 223. Subacute cutaneous lupus erythematosus, annular lesions.
Annular, red, scaly lesions may affect the trunk, especially the back, but also the arms and hands in SCLE. In a few patents, the malar rash or discoid lesions may be seen.

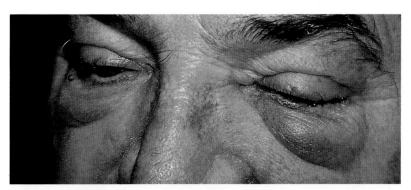

Figure 224. Dermatomyositis, periorbital edema. Dermatomyositis is a multi-system disorder affecting primarily the sun-exposed skin and muscle. Specific variants include juvenile (**Figure 124**), paraneoplastic, and amyopathic (lack of muscle involvement). Classic clinical signs include periorbital edema with a violaceous hue, a photodistributed eruption on the chest, upper back, and arms (see **Figure 475**), Gottron's papules (involvement of the knuckles), and periungual telangiectasia. Proximal muscle weakness is the classic systemic sign. There is a 15% incidence of cancer in adults but not in children (see **Figure 124**) under 16 years of age.

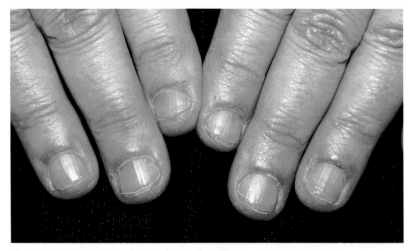

Figure 225. Dermatomyositis, periungual erythema. Periungual erythema and telangiectases occur in dermatomyositis (see **Figure 224**). Other collagen vascular diseases may be considered in differential diagnosis, e.g. systemic lupus erythematosus and scleroderma.

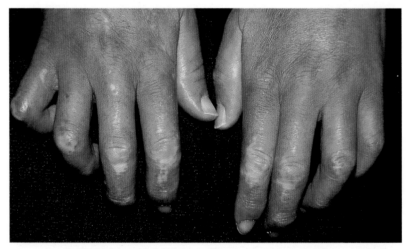

Figure 226. Scleroderma, sclerodactyly. Scleroderma (also known as systemic sclerosis) is characterized by progressive fibrosis of various organ systems, including the skin, heart, lung, kidney, and gastrointestinal tract. Diffuse thickening of the skin, associated with Raynaud's phenomenon, is typical. The term sclerodactyly refers to induration of the digits, and is illustrated here. The patient has extended her fingers as much as possible. Note the erythema and depigmentation over the digits. Ulceration of the fingertips and over the knuckles occurs and can be debilitating.

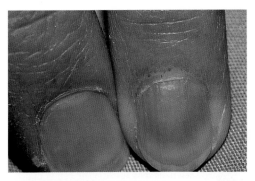

Figure 227. Scleroderma, nailfold capillaries.
Dilated and distorted capillary loops alternating with avascular areas occur in systemic sclerosis and dermatomyositis. Nailfold bleeding may occur. In this illustration, the finger on the left is normal.

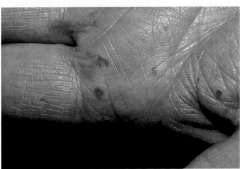

Figure 228. CREST syndrome, telangiectatic mats. **C**alcinosis cutis, **R**aynaud's phenomenon, **e**sophogeal dysfunction, **s**clerodactyly, and **t**elangiectases constitute the CREST syndrome, a variant of systemic scleroderma. Anticentromere antibodies are most characteristic of CREST but may also be found in systemic scleroderma patients.

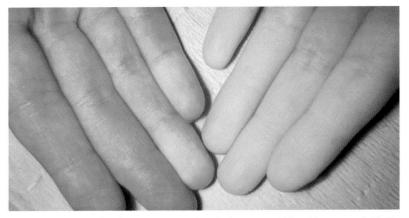

Figure 229. Raynaud's phenomenon.   Sharply demarcated blanching occurs initially, followed by cyanosis and subsequently hyperemia in Raynaud's phenomenon. One or multiple fingers may be affected, and cold exposure is the classic precipitating factor. Associations include collagen vascular disease, certain drugs, and arterial disease (e.g. thromboangiitis obliterans). When idiopathic, the term Raynaud's disease is used. (Courtesy of James Rasmussen, MD.)

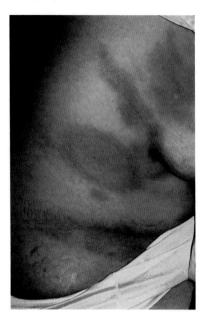

Figure 230. Morphea, also known as localized scleroderma, is a fibrotic condition of the skin in which indurated plaques develop. Some cases of morphea have been thought related to *Borrelia burgdorferi* infection, and *Borrelia* DNA has been detected in morphea by polymerase chain reaction. Women are more commonly affected, and multiple lesions may occur. Very rarely, patients may go on to develop systemic sclerosis. Morphea and lichen sclerosis may coexist. The center of a lesion of morphea is often ivory white with a border of erythema. The skin is indurated on palpation. The woman shown here has multiple lesions.
The one in the center of the picture is truncal, oval, with a central whitish hue and a red border.

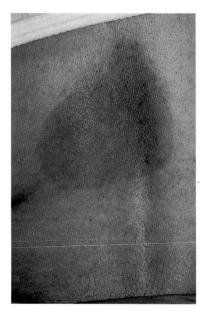

Figure 231. Atrophoderma of Pasini and Pierini.   Tan-to-light-brown atrophic patches varying in size from several centimeters to tens of centimeters on the back of a young woman are characteristic. This disease is closely related to, and at times may resemble, morphea. The darker color of the lesions compared with the skin adds to their appearance of being depressed. However, the lesions are atrophic, and the dermal atrophy of some of the lesions is so pronounced that a distinct 'drop off' at the edge is palpable. Serum antibodies to *Borrelia burgdorferi* have been reported positive in a significant proportion of patients. A zosteriform distribution and overlap cases with morphea and lichen sclerosis may occur.

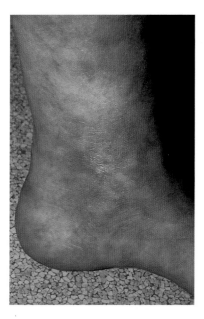

Figure 232. Linear scleroderma
(linear morphea) is a form of localized scleroderma characterized by sclerotic lesions distributed in a band-like pattern. Hypo- or hyperpigmented areas are often seen. It occurs most commonly on the leg but may also occur on the arm and forehead (where the term en coupe de sabre is used). A deep component with fixation to underlying structures may be present. Joint pains are common, and joint contractures caused by skin and tissue involvement may occur. Antinuclear antibody may be strongly positive. This woman's lesion extended the length of her inner leg.

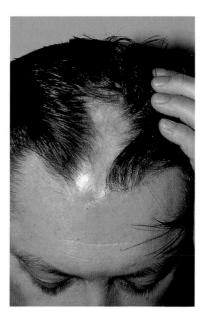

Figure 233. En coup de sabre.
A linear, indurated depression running vertically just to one side of the midline on the face is characteristic of en coup de sabre, a variant of morphea. The lesion may extend to the scalp causing an alopetic streak as shown here, or it may spread downward to involve the nose, lips, and chin.

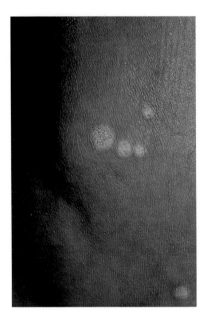

Figure 234. Lichen sclerosis, skin.
Lichen sclerosis (LS) is a chronic skin disorder of unknown etiology. It causes white plaques in the skin and is most common in the vulva. When it occurs on the skin, the trunk is the preferred site. Clinically, one sees ivory white papules and plaques with characteristic follicular plugging. This young girl's lesions occurred on the ankles. As with morphea, *Borrelia burgdorferi* DNA has been detected in LS by PCR. The significance of this is unknown.

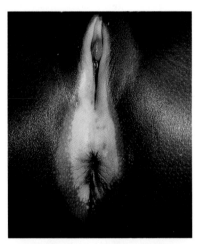

Figure 235. Lichen sclerosis, vulva.
Vulvar lichen sclerosis develops symmetrically about the vagina and rectum and tends to affect either prepubescent girls or perimenopausal women. Pruritus, burning pain, dyspareunia, dysuria, vaginal discharge, anal or genital bleeding, labial stenosis or fusion, constipation (especially in children), erosion, contraction, and squamous cell carcinoma may occur. The appearance in this patient is the classic 'hourglass' formed about the vagina and anus. (Courtesy of Michael O Murphy, MD)

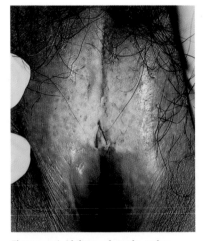

Figure 236. Lichen sclerosis, vulva.
This patient's lichen sclerosis is more limited, but with more hyperkeratotis.

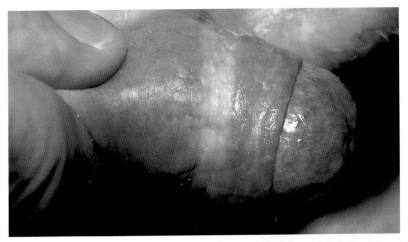

Figure 237. Balanitis xerotica obliterans is the term used for lichen sclerosis of the penis. This disease is a common cause of phimosis in boys. Squamous cell carcinoma may rarely occur. The glans and/or foreskin become white, smooth, and atrophic. Erosions, hemorrhage, decreased sensation of the glans, painful erections, and scarring with phimosis may occur.

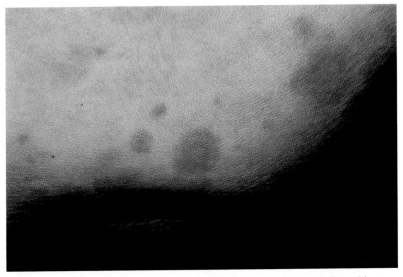

Figure 238. Still's disease is an evanescent rash that occurs in association with juvenile rheumatoid arthritis. It has been suggested that an infectious agent could trigger the disease in a genetically predisposed patient. The classic clinical appearance is an erythematous to salmon-colored urticarial rash occurring in the mid-day to evening on the trunk and proximal limbs. The rash often appears during the fever spikes. Fever and arthritis may be associated.

DRUG-RELATED DISORDERS

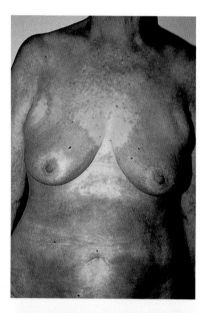

Figures 239 and 240. Maculopapular drug eruption. Erythematous macules and smooth papules scattered symmetrically across the trunk and elsewhere are characteristic. When faced with a patient on multiple medications, a book that lists specific drugs, the characteristic reaction pattern, and the likelihood of such an eruption, is invaluable. Compare the lesions in **Figure 240**, below, with the true target lesions of erythema multiforme (**Figure 412**).

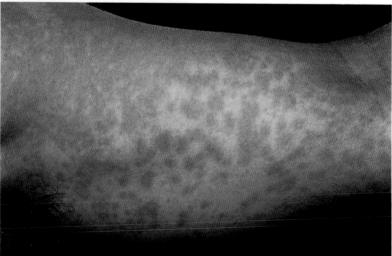

Figure 240. Maculopapular drug eruption. Individual erythematous, urticarial papules that coallesce into plaques is typical of the classic drug eruption. Onset is usually within one week of starting the offending agent. Compare with **Figure 412**.

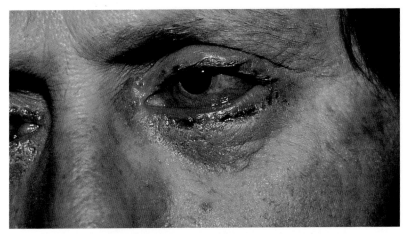

Figure 241. Stevens–Johnson syndrome (SJS) is a serious allergic reaction characterized by ocular and oral inflammation and diffuse skin reaction or erythema and bulla formation. A continuum exists between SJS and toxic epidermal necrolysis (**Figure 243**), with the amount of bulla formation and denudation differentiating the two. Inflammation, crusting and redness of the conjunctival, oral, and genital mucosa develop acutely. Headache, fever, and malaise also occur. Inability to eat, fluid loss, and infection are significant complications. Drugs are the most common cause (e.g. penicillins, phenytoin, sulfonamides), but an infection may be implicated.

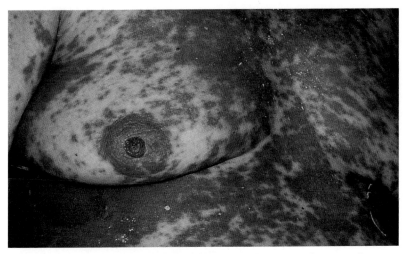

Figure 242. Stevens–Johnson syndrome. The rash of Stevens–Johnson syndrome may resemble the classic maculopapular drug rash but is often more dusky red, with areas of necrosis. Erosions, as illustrated below this woman's right breast, commonly occur.

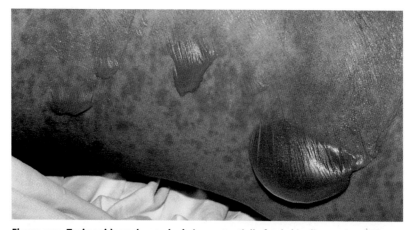

Figure 243. Toxic epidermal necrolysis is a potentially fatal skin disease in which much of the skin sloughs from the body. Ninety to 95% of cases are associated with drug use, the most common being antimicrobials (e.g. sulfonamides, penicillins, or cephalosporins), NSAIDs, and anticonvulsants. The patient degenerates from totally healthy to life-threateningly ill within a few days. A prodrome of malaise and fever is followed by diffuse erythema and edema of the skin. Bullae then develop, which enlarge until the epidermis sloughs off in large sheets.

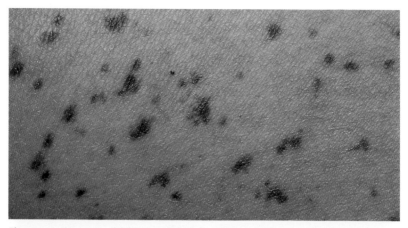

Figure 244. Hypersensitivity vasculitis is an allergic reaction, most commonly to a drug, but it has been reported in association with inflammatory bowel disease, large vessel vasculitis, malignancy, infection, cryoglobulins, and collagen vascular disease. A shower of purpuric lesions, both palpable and non-palpable, concentrated on the legs is seen clinically. Associated symptoms include fever, malaise, nausea, and arthralgias. Often, this eruption resolves before a work-up can be completed. (Compare with true target lesions of erythema multiforme, **Figure 412.**)

Figure 245. Acute exanthematous pustulosis, also called toxic pustuloderma, is an unusual pustular allergic reaction, usually to a drug. The onset is typically within a day of exposure to the offending agent. Clinically, one sees a rapidly developing non-follicular pustular eruption on diffusely erythematous skin. The pustules are sterile.

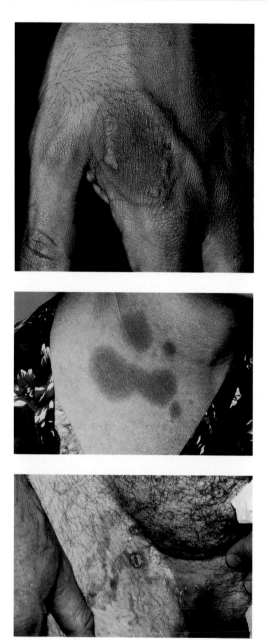

Figure 246. Fixed drug eruption, solitary.
Single or multiple, dusky-red, round or oval lesions occurring repeatedly in a fixed site after each exposure to the offending drug are characteristic. Crusting or blistering, as shown here, may occur. Typical drugs to consider include tetracycline, sulfa drugs, ampicillin, and phenolphthalein.

Figure 247. Fixed drug eruption, multiple.
With each subsequent exposure to the drug, the initial lesion may increase in size, and additional lesions may develop.

Figure 248. Corticosteroid-induced striae and erosions. Topical steroids are tremendously beneficial in the treatment of skin disease. However, the inappropriate use of high potency topical steroids can lead to atrophy, striae, and even ulceration as shown here. The face and flexural areas are particularly prone to these side effects. This patient was using a combination of clotrimazole and betamethasone valerate for many months for a non-specific groin rash.

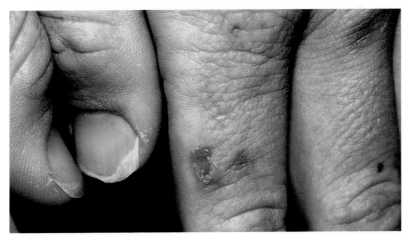

Figure 249. Pseudoporphyria.   The term pseudoporphyria is used when porphyria cutanea tarda (PCT)-like lesions arise in the setting of normal porphyrin levels. It usually results from the combination of a weak photosensitizing drug and sun exposure (but it may also occur in the setting of hemodialysis). Typical drugs include sulfonamides, dapsone, furosemide, nalidixic acid, naproxen, ibuprofen, pyridoxone, nabumetone, fluoroquinolone antibiotics, or tetracycline. Ultraviolet exposure is critical for the development of pseudoporphyria, and patients may either be spending significant time in the sun, or visiting a tanning booth. As with PCT, vesicles, erosions, and fragility on the dorsa of the hands is characteristic, although hypertrichosis or hyperpigmentation are typically absent. An extremely common offending agent is naproxen, which is an over-the-counter medication widely used for pain control. The patient shown had been receiving naproxen for 8 months.

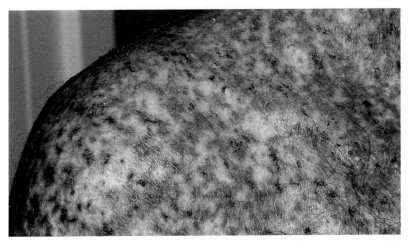

Figure 250. 5-Fluorouracil reaction.   5-Fluorouracil is commonly used to treat actinic keratoses. Tremendous erosive lesions, crusting, and inflammation develop during use. Intravenous 5-fluorouracil, as used to treat cancer, can induce these changes, which was how this treatment for actinic keratoses was initially discovered.

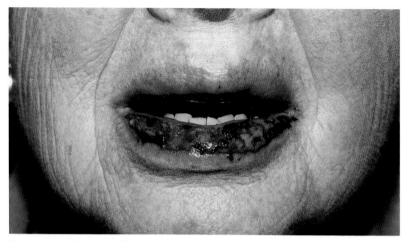

Figure 251. 5-Fluorouracil reaction. 5-Fluorouracil is commonly used to treat actinic cheilitis. Tremendous erosive changes will occur here as well, but the lip will heal dramatically well.

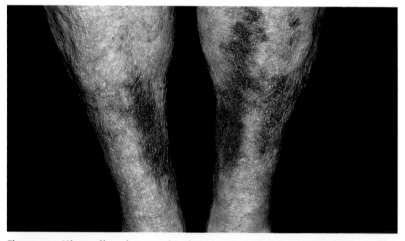

Figure 252. Minocycline pigmentation, legs. Minocycline has been used for years to treat acne, but recently its uses have been expanded to other inflammatory diseases, e.g. rheumatoid arthritis. Chronic use can lead to deposition of minocycline–iron (or other compound) complexes that give a bluish color to the skin, eyes, or nails. This patient had been treated with minocycline for years for her rheumatoid arthritis. The color changes are cosmetic only, and she elected to continue treatment.

ECZEMATOUS DERMATOSES

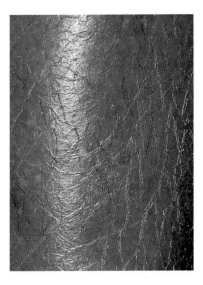

Figure 253. Xerosis, legs. The skin may be thought of as a wet sponge covered by a thin oil membrane. When the surface oil is depleted, the sponge dries out. An atopic background, dry, cold weather, frequent water contact, advanced age, and irritants predispose to dry skin, also known as xerosis. The shins are commonly affected.

Figure 254. Asteatotic eczema, legs. When the skin's superficial water barrier is lost, the underlying skin dries out and may become inflamed. The legs of elderly people in the winter months are commonly affected. The skin appears erythematous and cracked with wide but superficial fissures.

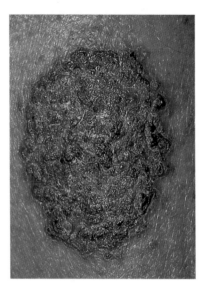

Figure 255. Nummular eczema.
The appearance of this lesion is *not* that of ringworm (**Figure 330**). The redness and inflammation is uniformly distributed throughout. An 'active border' is not seen. Typically, as in this patient, multiple lesions tend to erupt on the arms and legs. Pruritus is usually significant. Risk factors include excessive bathing (e.g. more than 10 minutes), other prolonged water exposure (e.g. regular swimming), and dry, cold air.

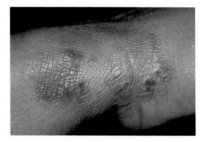

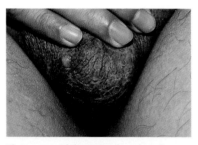

Figure 256. Lichen simplex chronicus.
Scratching is never good. It opens the skin up to infection, prevents healing, and may induce lesions through Köbnerization. It also hides characteristic changes of any primary lesion, making the physician's work that much harder. Lichen simplex chronicus is a term used to describe thickened skin that has resulted from chronic rubbing and scratching. Illustrated here are two chronic, lichenified, excoriated plaques in a patient with atopic dermatitis. Accentuation of the skin lines (lichenification) is seen.

Figure 257. Lichen simplex chronicus
may occur virtually anywhere, but common sites include the ankle, shin, scrotum, vulva, nape and side of the neck. It is often less threatening and more helpful when trying to elicit a history of chronic scratching to ask the patient, 'Does it itch?' rather than asking, 'Do you scratch?'.

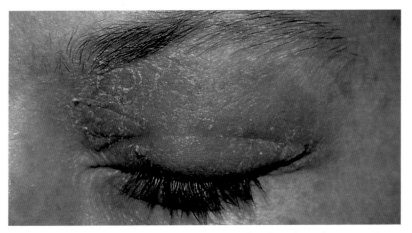

Figure 258. Eyelid dermatitis.   Chronic redness and scaling about the eyes are very common, especially in women. The most common causes are allergic contact, irritant contact, atopic, and seborrheic dermatitis. Work-up should include inquiry into the patient's occupation (e.g. any airborne matter, sawdust), use of potential allergens (e.g. nail polish, makeup, eyeliner, eye drops), a complete skin examination (to look for signs of atopic dermatitis, psoriasis, or seborrheic dermatitis), and patch testing.

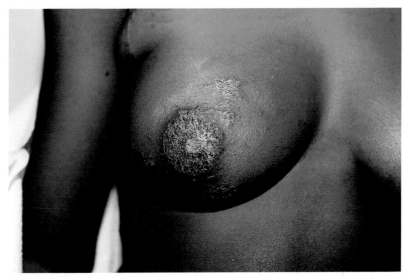

Figure 259. Nipple dermatitis.   The nipples commonly become eczematous in both men and women, probably because of friction with the bra and/or clothing. Scratching aggravates the problem and can induce a vicious cycle.

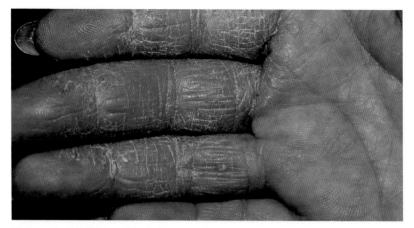

Figure 260. Hand dermatitis, irritant. Irritant contact dermatitis represents irritation and inflammation of the skin arising from exposure to (usually chemical) stimuli. A specific immune-mediated allergic reaction is excluded. It may occur almost anywhere on the body, but the hands are commonly affected because they often come in contact with potential irritants. In fact, chronic hand dermatitis poses a significant problem for the patient, physician. and employer. Inquiry should be made regarding the patient's occupation, hobbies, the frequency of hand washing, and exposure to chemicals or irritants. Allergic contact dermatitis should be excluded. This woman developed an irritant hand dermatitis soon after having her first baby.

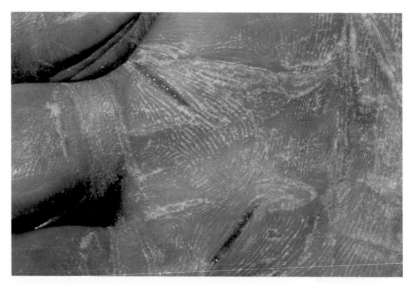

Figure 261. Hyperkeratotic eczema is a relatively common type of eczema of the hands in adults. It often affects men and is a significant cause of time off work. Diffuse, thickened, fissured hyperkeratosis of the palms is seen. Patch testing and the potassium hydroxide examination to exclude other causes are important. Fissuring, as illustrated here, can be painful.

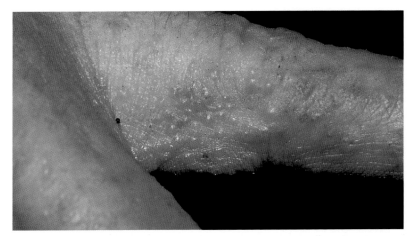

Figure 262. Pompholyx, vesicles. Tiny 'tapioca' vesicles of the sides of the fingers but also fingertips, palms, and soles occur in this condition, also called dyshidrotic eczema. Areas may become red, scaly, and weeping, and the patient usually complains of intense itching. A mild form may occur in which small vesicles rupture to form enlarging collarettes of scale. A severe form may occur with large palmar and plantar bullae.

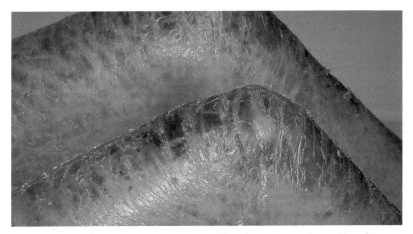

Figure 263. Exfoliative erythroderma is a term used to describe the patient whose body is covered from head to toe with erythema and variable scale. This presentation may be caused by various entities including a medication, psoriasis, atopic dermatitis, pityriasis rubra pilaris, and most importantly cutaneous T-cell lymphoma. The initial work-up for patients who have no obvious cause includes a thorough history and physical exam, complete blood count, and skin biopsy. If these are unrevealing, lymph node biopsy or CT scan may be done.

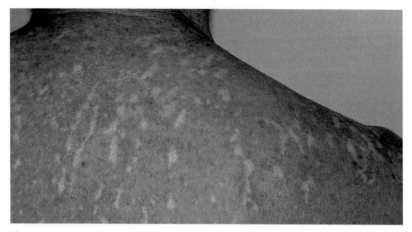

Figure 264. Neurotic excoriations. Various disorders, including trichotillomania, neurotic excoriations, and dermatitis artefacta, are facticial or self-inflicted. The term neurotic excoriations describes the patient who picks and scratches the skin usually in response to anxiety or stress in the absence of a primary dermatologic disorder. The patient, usually a woman, may be either totally aware or totally unaware of the cause of her skin changes. The upper back and the flexural surfaces of the extremities are most commonly affected. Linear (as shown here) or round-to-oval white scars accumulate over time. A primary dermatosis should be excluded as well as delusions of parasitosis.

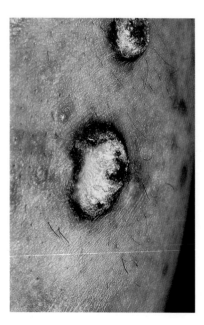

Figure 265. Prurigo nodularis. Chronic scratching can eventually result in the formation of nodules.

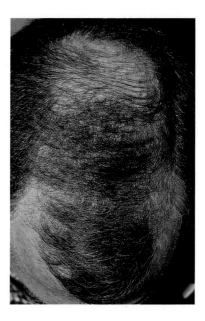

Figure 266. Androgenic alopecia, male. A young man in his 20s or 30s may become very distressed and seek medical help because of hair loss at the vertex and bilaterally along the frontotemporal areas. Individual hairs become smaller, and the hairline recedes. Later, the forehead becomes taller and, finally, all terminal hair may be lost from the forehead to the vertex. The early onset of androgenic alopecia puts the patient at increased risk of ischemic heart disease.

General work-up for hair loss in a woman. There is no figure for this condition because the majority of women who seek medical attention for thinning hair seem normal on examination. This is because a significant portion of the hair must be lost before the change is clinically apparent. The history and a physical and laboratory examination should exclude telogen effluvium, thyroid disease, hormonal abnormalities, drug-induced alopecia, and low iron. If no cause is found, the diagnosis of androgenic alopecia is made.

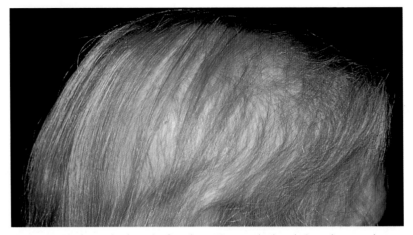

Figure 267. Androgenic alopecia, female.   Women who lose hair as they age do so in a pattern different from men. The hairline is preserved, but thinning develops from the frontal hairline to the vertex. A family history may or may not be found.

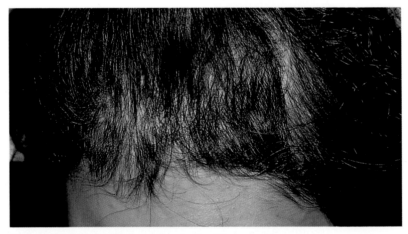

Figure 268. Telogen effluvium refers to the diffuse shedding of hair 2–3 months after a stressful event. Causes include chronic systemic diseases (e.g. liver failure, renal failure, cancer), severe psychological stress, surgery and/or anesthesia, crash dieting, acute physical stress (e.g. high fever, severe bleeding), and giving birth. The patient presents with a several week history of increased hair loss as seen on her pillow, brush, or in the shower. She may pull at her hair in the office, showing how easily the hairs are removed. If the stress is removed, normal hair regrowth is expected.

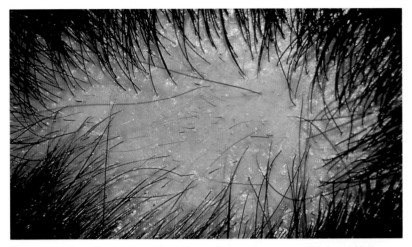

Figure 269. Alopecia areata, scalp. The sudden and near complete loss of hair in one or more circular patches is characteristic of alopecia areata, a disease that affects children and young adults preferentially. The cause is unknown. Short, blunt-ended hairs, tapered at the base (exclamation point hairs), may be seen near the margin of the alopecia.

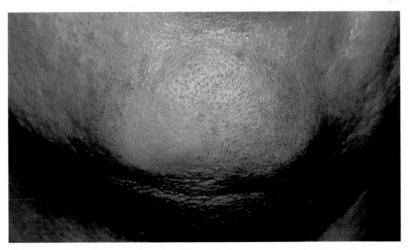

Figure 270. Alopecia areata, beard. The scalp is most commonly affected by alopecia areata, but loss can occur in the eyebrows, eyelashes, beard, and elsewhere.

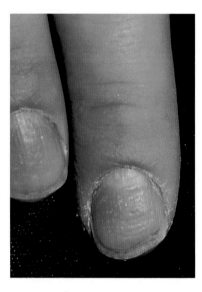

Figure 271. Alopecia areata, pits, nails.
Pits may occur in the nail in a uniform grid-like pattern.

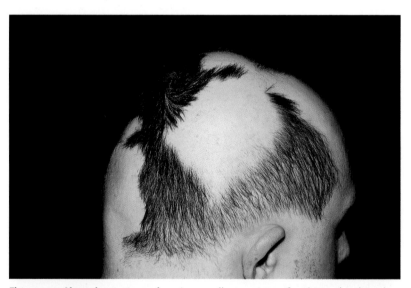

Figure 272. Alopecia areata, scalp.   In a small percentage of patients, the alopecia becomes more widespread.

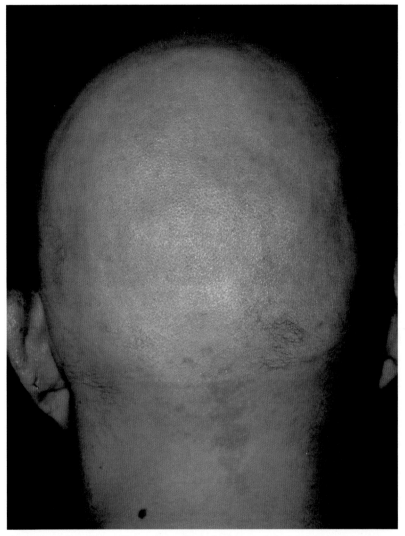

Figure 273. Alopecia totalis, scalp. When all of the scalp hair is lost in alopecia areata, the term alopecia totalis is used. When all hair everywhere is lost, the term alopecia universalis is used. The physician must be sensitive to the emotional and psychological distress that may accompany the loss of all one's hair. (Erythema nuchae is also seen here.)

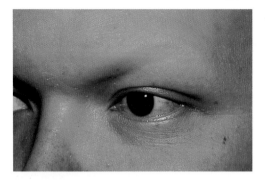

Figure 274. Alopecia universalis. Note the loss of both eyebrow hair and the eyelashes.

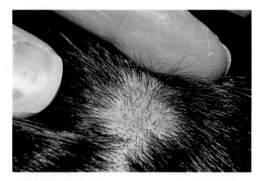

Figure 275. Trichotillomania, localized. In trichotillomania, hair loss occurs secondary to pulling or other manipulation by the patient. Young girls are most commonly affected. Parent–child issues or psychological problems may be associated. One characteristic sign is that the remaining hairs are not uniform in length. Often, a peripheral collar of normal hair is seen along the hairline. The nails may be dystrophic from onychophagia causing a similar appearance to that of alopecia areata, but pits are not seen.

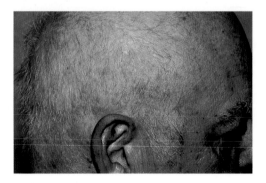

Figure 276. Anagen effluvium. A toxic insult to the body can preferentially affect the hair bulb because of its active metabolism. Diffuse hair loss can result and is called anagen effluvium. Cancer chemotherapeutic drugs are the most common offenders. Permanent damage is not done, and hair regrowth is expected if the insult is removed.

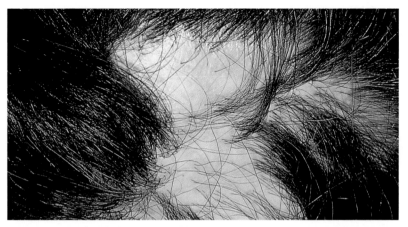

Figure 277. Pseudopelade is an idiopathic, scarring alopecia characterized by round to oval areas of hair loss like 'footprints in the snow'. There may be perifollicular erythema early and moderate atrophy in late stages, but no crust, scale, or follicular hyperkeratosis is seen. Most patients are women. The course is chronic with slow progression. The key differential diagnoses are cutaneous lupus erythematosus and lichen planopilaris.

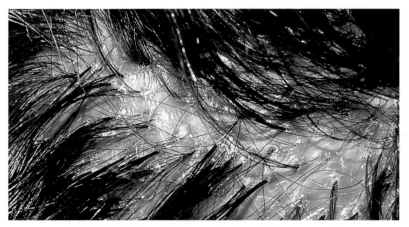

Figure 278. Tufted folliculitis.   Tufted hairs or polytrichia forming in the setting of chronic *Staphylococcus aureus* infection of the scalp, acne keloidalis nuchae, folliculitis decalvans, or dissecting cellulitis of the scalp, is characteristic. This disease is not a single entity but a clinical finding in the setting of various inflammatory alopecias. The tufts of hair probably form through compaction by scars and inflammation.

HIV-RELATED DERMATOSES

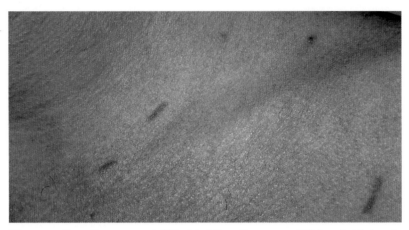

Figure 279. Kaposi's sarcoma.   HIV-related Kaposi's sarcoma (KS) is a viral-induced vascular malignancy in HIV-positive patients. The virus has been identified as human herpes virus 8 and has been found in all forms of KS, including HIV-associated KS, classic KS, and endemic KS, as well as body-cavity lymphomas associated with HIV. HIV-related Kaposi's sarcoma usually presents as an asymptomatic, erythematous macule that later becomes raised and violaceous. Larger truncal lesions tend to be ovoid, following lines of cleavage as illustrated here.

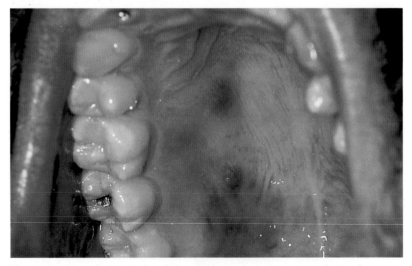

Figure 280. Kaposi's sarcoma, palate.   KS lesions are common on the trunk, extremities, and oral cavity (where the palate is preferred).

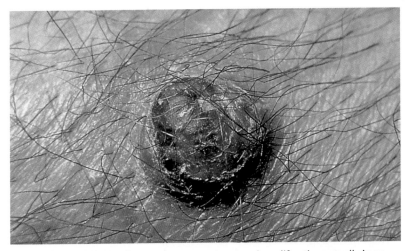

Figure 281. Bacillary angiomatosis represents an angioproliferation, usually in an immunocompromised host, caused by either *Bartonella henselae* (formerly *Rochalimaea henselae*) or *B. quintana* (formerly *R. quintana*) and that is acquired most commonly from a cat bite, scratch, or lick or possibly from cat fleas. Pyogenic granuloma-like lesions, reddish-purple papulonodules, and/or subcutaneous nodules in a patient with AIDS are characteristic. Systemic symptoms (e.g. fever, chills, malaise) as well as systemic involvement (especially of the liver) may occur. (Courtesy of Caroline Thornton, MD.)

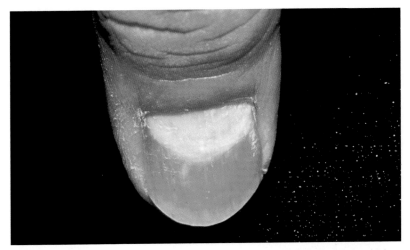

Figure 282. Proximal subungual onychomycosis is a rare type of infection in which the fungus invades the area under the nail via the proximal nail fold. This type of infection is most common in the HIV-positive population. Clinically, one sees a proximal whitish discoloration under the nail. *Trichophyton rubrum* is the most common organism.

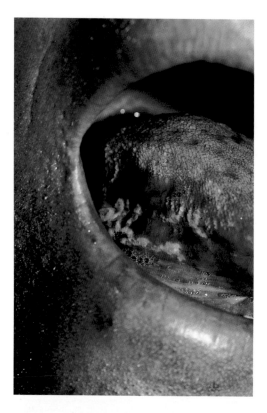

Figure 283. Oral hairy leukoplakia is a common, benign disorder of the oral cavity of patients with HIV that has been associated with Epstein–Barr virus (EBV) infection. White, verrucous, corrugated plaques on the sides of the tongue in an HIV-positive patient are characteristic. The lesions are usually asymptomatic. Occasionally, the dorsum of the tongue, buccal mucosa and/or palate may be involved. Lesions on the pharynx and esophagus have been described. Occasionally patients with other types of immunosuppression may be affected (e.g. renal transplant patients). The term pseudo hairy leukoplakia is used for patients with clinically similar lesions who are HIV negative, immunocompetent, and where no EBV is found.

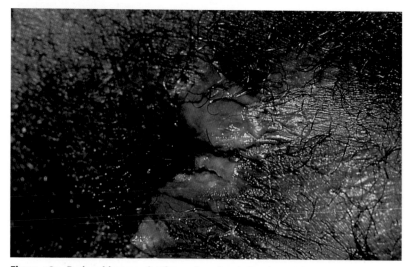

Figure 284. Perianal herpes simplex. A perianal ulcer in an HIV-positive patient represents a herpes simplex infection until proven otherwise.

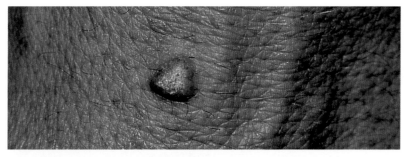

Figure 285. Herpes zoster/verruciform lesions.   Multiple, disseminated hyperkeratotic, verrucous papules and plaques in an HIV-positive patient may represent chronic infection by the varicella zoster virus.

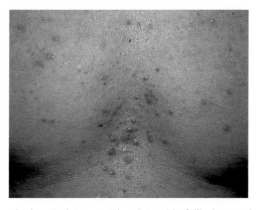

Figure 286. Eosinophilic folliculitis is a common itchy follicular disease that tends to present in HIV patients late in their disease who have low CD4 counts. It may also occur in patients being treated for hematologic malignancy, including 2–3 months after bone marrow transplantation. The cause is not known, but it has been suggested that an autoimmune process against the sebocyte or a constituent of sebum is the cause. Chronic pruritic, follicular papules of the trunk, neck, and arms in an HIV-positive patient are characteristic. Occasionally, one can see a few intact pustules. Intense scratching often leads to bleeding, crusting, and eroded papules. A bacterial folliculitis caused by *Staphylococcus aureus* or *Pseudomonas aeruginosa* should be excluded.

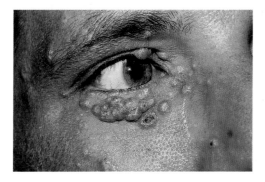

Figure 287. Molluscum contagiosum, periorbital area.   Innumerable flesh-colored papules of the face are common in HIV-positive patients. Papules in the beard area may be spread through shaving. The presence of organisms in clinically normal adjacent skin may explain its resistance to therapy. (See also **Figures 91, 92** and **350** for molluscum contagiosum infection in non-HIV patients.)

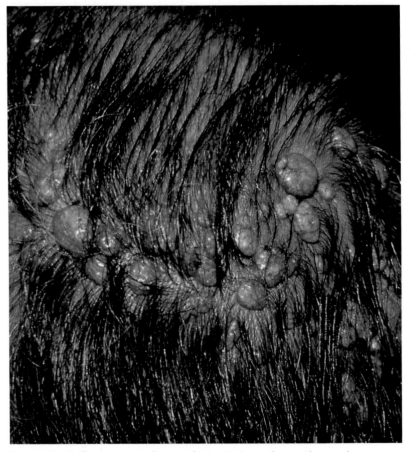

Figure 288. Molluscum contagiosum, giant.   At times, the papules may become large, presenting a difficult therapeutic problem.

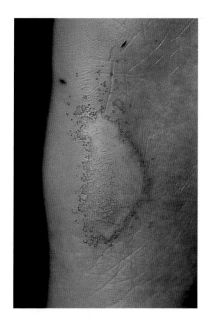

Figure 289. Pitted keratolysis is a superficial infection of the skin confined to the stratum corneum and caused by the bacterium *Kytococcus sedentarius*. Multiple 1–2 mm pits in a teenager wearing footwear for prolonged periods with sweating is typical. Malodour and sliminess of the skin occur in most cases. The pressure-bearing areas, such as the ventral aspect of the toe, the ball of the foot, and the heel are typical sites for the onset of lesions. Lesions are rarely seen on the non-pressure-bearing locations.

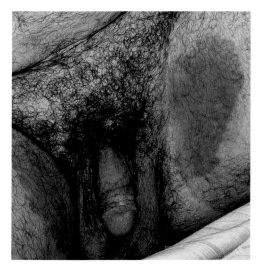

Figure 290. Erythrasma is a superficial infection of the flexures of the skin caused by the bacterium *Corynebacterium minutissimum*. *Corynebacterium afermentans* has also been reported. Red-brown patches, commonly of the groin or axilla, with distinct borders and little to no scale occur.

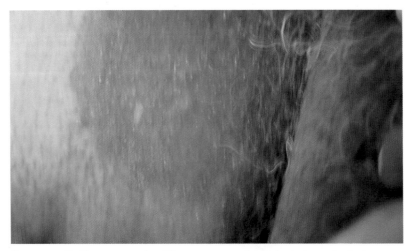

Figure 291. Erythrasma, coral red fluorescence. *Corynebacterium minutissimum* creates a water-soluble porphyrin that fluoresces coral pink under Wood's light examination. This finding may be absent if the patient has recently bathed.

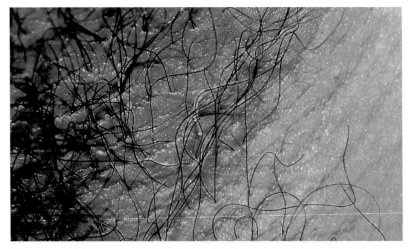

Figure 292. Trichomycosis axillaris. Yellow, red, or black attachments on the hair as a result of bacterial colonization occurs in trichomycosis axillaris. *Corynebacterium tenuis* is one of the bacteria which has been identified.

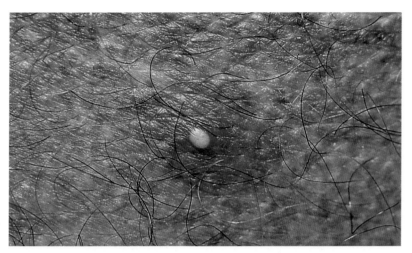

Figure 293. Staphylococcal folliculitis, pustule. Multiple follicular pustules scattered on the trunk may represent a bacterial folliculitis. Excoriations may mask the primary pustule. Culture establishes the diagnosis and can indicate the appropriate antibiotic choice.

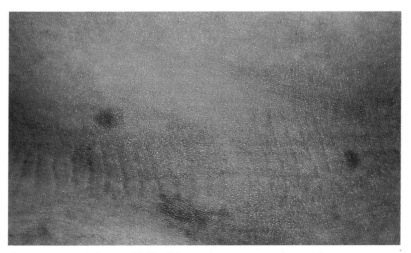

Figure 294. Staphylococcal folliculitis, erythematous papules. Often, staphylococcal folliculitis lesions are deep-seated and appear only as erythematous papules.

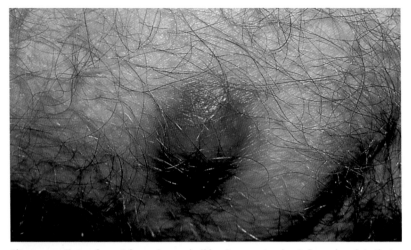

Figure 295. Furuncle. A furuncle or a boil begins as a tender, inflamed nodule that usually becomes fluctuant, points, and ruptures.

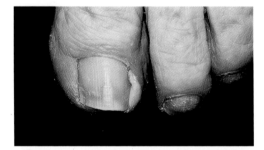

Figure 296. Paronychia, acute. Acute paronychia is often caused by *Staphylococcus aureus*. (See **Figure 460**.)

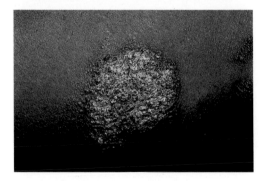

Figure 297. Blastomycosis-like pyoderma is an uncommon manifestation of a chronic cutaneous bacterial infection. Verrucous, hyperkeratotic plaque or plaques that resemble blastomycosis are seen (compare with **Figure 339**). *Staphylococcus aureus* and *Streptococcus* species are the most common pathogens, but *Pseudomonas* species has been reported. Alcoholism, diabetes, and trauma have been reported as predisposing factors.

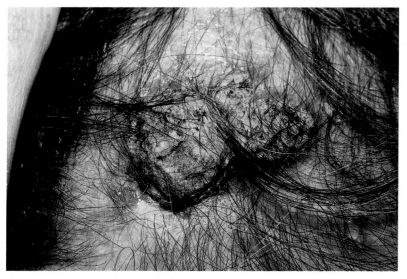

Figure 298. Bacterial infection of the scalp. An ulcer or erosion of the scalp of an older individual (e.g. after curettage and electrodesiccation of a basal cell carcinoma) is prone to secondary infection by both Gram-positive and Gram-negative bacteria. A solid crust overlying greenish pus is typical of a Gram-negative infection and is illustrated here.

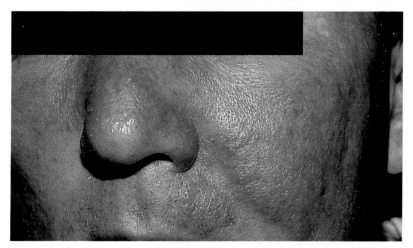

Figure 299. Erysipelas, face. Cellulitis is a term describing an expanding bacterial infection of the skin. The term erysipelas is used to describe a specific subset caused by the beta-hemolytic *Streptococcus* species. Clinically, one sees the acute onset of a bright red, warm, spreading, edematous plaque. The cheek (as shown here) is a common location. Fever or chills may accompany the rash, and pustules or skin breakdown may occur.

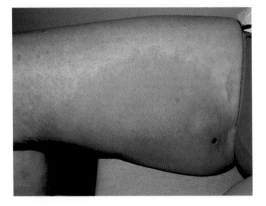

Figure 300. Erysipelas, leg.
The acute onset of a warm, erythematous, edematous plaque that each day enlarges several to many centimeters is characteristic. Fever and chills or more severe skin changes (e.g. purpura, bullae, postbullous ulceration, necrosis, hypoesthesia, or fluctuance) may suggest necrotizing fasciitis or pyomyositis. Risk factors include impaired venous or lymphatic return, diabetes mellitus, atherosclerosis, NSAID use and a pre-existing open lesion.

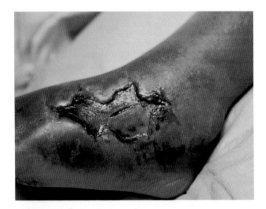

Figure 301. Necrotizing fasciitis. The so-called flesh eating bacteria—group A beta-hemolytic *Streptococcus* species—can cause significant tissue destruction rapidly. This 32-year-old woman developed pain, erythema, and swelling of the foot followed by necrotic ulceration over a week. There was no history of trauma. (Courtesy of Roger Bitar, MD.)

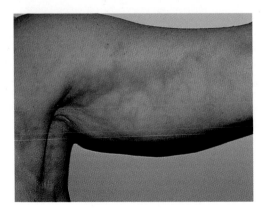

Figure 302. Lymphangitic streaking. This woman, postmastectomy, developed cellulitis of the forearm with subsequent lymphangitic streaking along the defective lymphatic system.

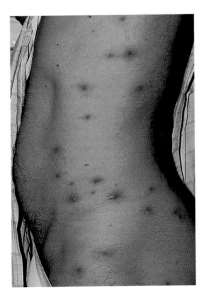

Figure 303. Hot-tub folliculitis.
The typical patient with hot-tub folliculitis develops multiple pustules on top of urticarial bases scattered on the trunk and/or buttocks several days after using a hot tub contaminated by the Gram-negative bacterium *Pseudomonas aeruginosa*. Prolonged hydration and occlusion of the skin (e.g. by a tight bathing suit) promote infection.

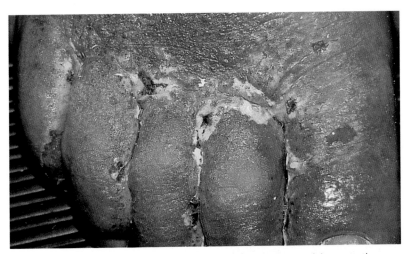

Figure 304. Gram-negative toe-web infection. Dermatophytes of the toe-web space may produce penicillin and streptomycin-like substances that allow Gram-negative bacteria to overgrow. The distal foot and toes become swollen, inflamed and malodorous. *Proteus* species and *Pseudomonas* species are often found. The affected patient often wears shoes most of the day.

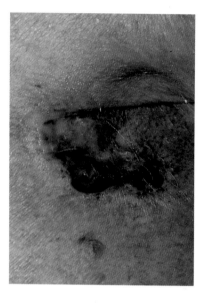

Figure 305. Ecthyma gangrenosum. One or multiple, well-defined areas of necrosis and ulceration may develop as a manifestation of *Pseudomonas aeruginosa* infection. The initial lesion is often a bulla or hemorrhagic pustule. The classic adult with ecthyma gangrenosum is a very ill, immunocompromised patient in the intensive care unit. Infants may be affected in the diaper area.

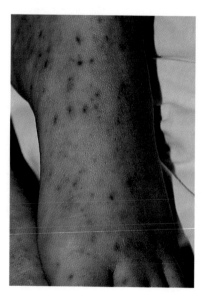

Figure 306. Neisseria meningitidis, distal purpura. The classic patient is a child or teenager who acutely develops severe headache, nausea, vomiting, and fever. Meningeal symptoms may occur, and the mental state may deteriorate to disorientation or even coma. Hypotensive shock and death may rapidly ensue. A petechial rash, often on the extensor hands, arms, and feet, is characteristic.

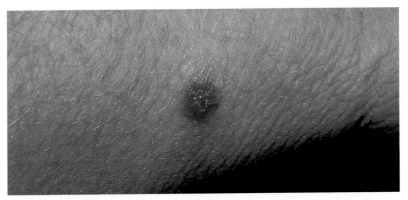

Figure 307. Cat scratch disease, papule at cat scratch. A scratch on the hand or arm by a cat followed weeks later by painful lymphadenopathy that may suppurate is characteristic. The causative organism is *Bartonella henselae*. Patients are likely to have a kitten which has scratched them, licked them on the face, or bitten them, or to have a kitten with fleas.

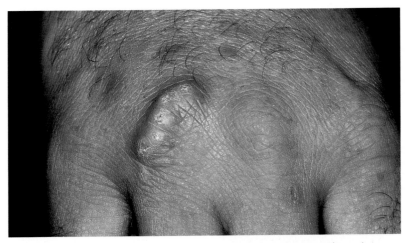

Figure 308. Atypical mycobacterial infection. Non-tuberculous mycobacteria are called atypical mycobacteria. Although they are quite prevalent in nature, infection is relatively rare. Immunocompromised hosts may develop systemic infection, whereas infection in a normal host is usually localized. The organisms that are most commonly encountered in clinical practice, *Mycobacterium avium*, *M. intracellulare*, *M. kansasii*, *M. fortuitum*, *M. abscessus*, and *M. chelonae*, are frequently found in water sources and soil. *Mycobacterium marinum* is a common cause of atypical mycobacterial infection in patients who have contact with a swimming pool, fish tank, or any hobbies or occupations that bring the patient in contact with fish. The disease is also known as a swimming pool or fish tank granuloma. If acquired from an aquarium, the dominant hand is typically affected. If acquired from a pool, any site of trauma may be affected. Typically, one sees a violaceous, crusted, or hyperkeratotic papulonodule on the dorsal surface of the hand or finger, often over a knuckle.

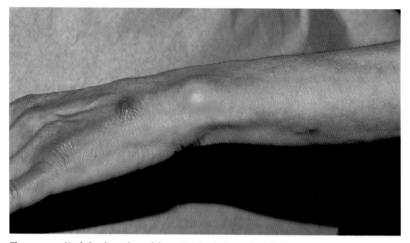

Figure 309. Nodular lymphangitis.   Tender inflamed nodules, progressing up the arm and originating from a traumatic injury to the hand—so-called sporotrichoid spread—are characteristic of nodular lymphangitis, also called lymphocutaneous syndrome. The most common atypical mycobacterium to spread in a sporotrichoid fashion is *Mycobacterium marinum*, as shown here. Other infectious agents that may be found include *Leishmania* species, *Nocardia brasiliensis*, *Francisella tularensis* and, of course, *Sporothrix schenckii*.

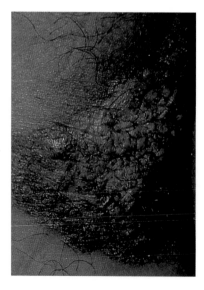

Figure 310. Tuberculosis verrucosa cutis. A chronic, warty plaque on the hand, knees, ankles, or buttocks (as shown here) is characteristic of this infection caused by *Mycobacterium tuberculosis*. Inoculation may have occurred from the patient's own saliva, another's saliva (e.g. sitting on spit), or from work (e.g. a pathologist with a prosector's wart).

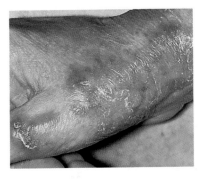

Figure 311. Lupus vulgaris represents an infection by *Mycobacterium tuberculosis* in a patient with moderate to high immunity and may have developed from local inoculation, lymphatic or hematogenous spread. Clinically, one sees a hyperkeratotic, crusted, granulomatous plaque or plaques on the face or elsewhere. An apple jelly color is seen on diascopy (pressure to remove the blood with a glass slide). (Courtesy of Christopher EM Griffiths, MD.)

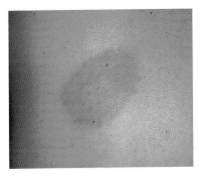

Figure 312. Erythema migrans is the skin manifestation of Lyme disease, a tick-borne illness caused by *Borrelia burgdorferi*. A red papule or macule which rapidly enlarges to form an annular lesion within a month of, and at the site of, a tick bite is characteristic. The primary lesion may also be an urticarial plaque without central clearing or have a central dusky purpuric or necrotic appearance. (Courtesy of Daniel K Frum, MD.)

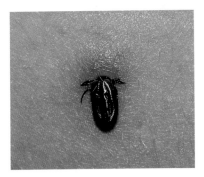

Figure 313. Tick bite by *Ixodes pacificus*. The vector for Lyme disease is the *Ixodes* tick. It appears that the tick must be attached for at least 24 hours to infect. Methods that help prevent Lyme disease include avoiding endemic, wooded areas, applying insect repellent, wearing long pants and long-sleeved shirts, tucking pants into socks, and checking regularly for ticks, removing them promptly if found.

See also bullous impetigo (**Figure 134**).

SUPERFICIAL FUNGAL INFECTIONS

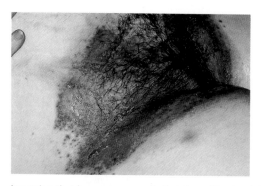

Figure 314. Candidiasis is infection by the yeast *Candida*. This infection may occur in various locations that may remain moist, e.g. the vagina, groin, inframammary fold, the mouth (**Figure 317**), the penis (candida balanitis, **Figure 318**), and the web spaces (erosio interdigitalis blastomycetica). At times, the initial condition is intertrigo that becomes secondarily infected by *Candida* species. The skin is inflamed and red. Scaling may or may not be present. Obese women with large breasts exposed to hot humid climates are most commonly affected.

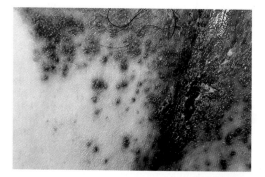

Figure 315. Candidiasis, satellite pustules. In candidiasis, there are often pustules scattered 1–3 cm beyond the edge of the erythema—so called satellite pustules.

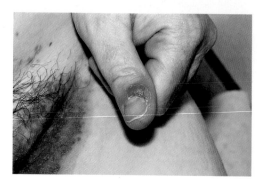

Figure 316. Candidal paronychia. The same patient as in **Figures 314** and **315** had a candidal paronychia.

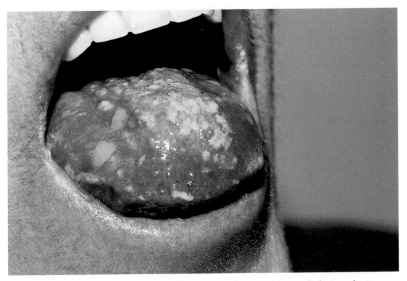

Figure 317. Thrush. In adults, HIV infection, corticosteroid use, diabetes, dentures, old age, and any cause of depressed cell-mediated immunity are risk factors for candidiasis of the oral mucosa. White, creamy papules and plaques occur, and the underlying mucosa may be red and inflamed. Healthy infants, especially those that are premature, and children on antibiotics may also be affected.

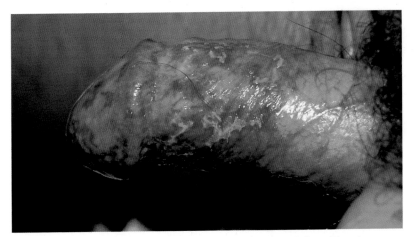

Figure 318. Candida balanitis. Bright red erythema initially, followed by minute pustules on the glans penis is characteristic. Uncircumcised men are at higher risk. A white, creamy coating may develop. The organism may have been obtained from the patient's own gastrointestinal tract or a sexual partner's genitals or anus. In severe cases, dysuria, pain with intercourse, and phimosis may occur.

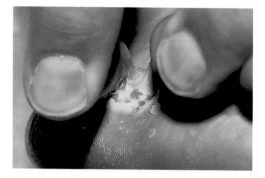

Figure 319. Tinea pedis, interdigital. Relatively asymptomatic, uncomplicated scaling of the web space is characteristic of simple dermatophyte infection. The web between the 4th and 5th toes is most often affected. When a mixed infection of dermatophyte and bacteria develops, the area may become white, macerated, and malodorous.

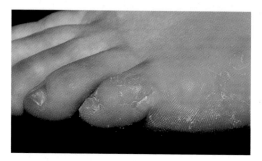

Figure 320. Tinea pedis. Redness and scaling of the web spaces initially but later over some or all of the sole (moccasin distribution) are characteristic. Potassium hydroxide examination or culture is confirmatory.

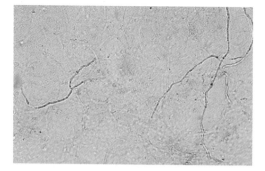

Figure 321. Potassium hydroxide examination. Virtually any relatively flat, scaly lesion should raise the suspicion of fungal infection. The potassium hydroxide examination is invaluable because of its ease, simplicity, and quick results. Abundant scale is scraped onto a microscopic slide with a blade and covered with a coverslip. KOH 10–20% with or without dimethyl sulfoxide (DMSO) is added. Fungal hyphae stand out as linear, branching, septate filaments of uniform width. (Courtesy of Terence C O'Grady, MD.)

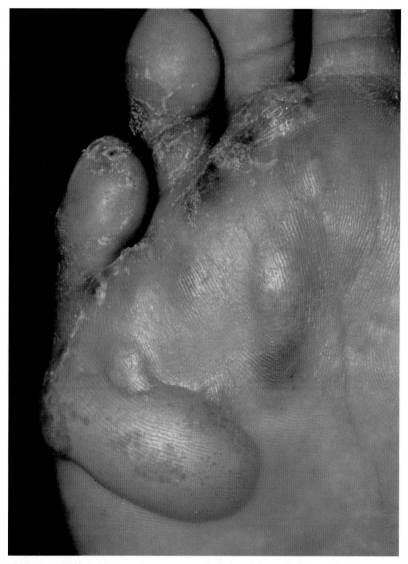

Figure 322. Bullous tinea.   An acute eruption of vesicles or bullae on the sole or sides of the foot is characteristic of bullous tinea. The lesions are usually pruritic and rarely painful. Often *Trichophyton mentagrophytes* is the causative fungus. The method of bulla formation appears to be the same as that for allergic contact dermatitis.

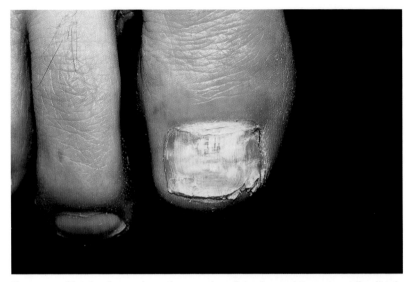

Figure 323. Distal subungual onychomycosis. Fungal organisms enter at the distal edge of the nail bed. Subungual debris accumulates, lifting the nail and causing onycholysis. Invasion of the nail plate causes it to thicken and turn yellow, brown, or white. The causative agent is usually a dermatophyte but one may also find a yeast (e.g. *Candida* species) or a mold (e.g. *Aspergillus* species).

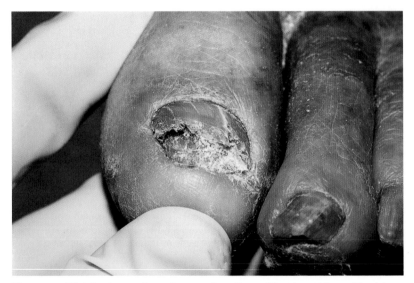

Figure 324. Distal subungual onychomycosis. The nail has been trimmed back to show the crumbly, subungual debris which is loaded with hyphae. This material is excellent for culturing the fungus.

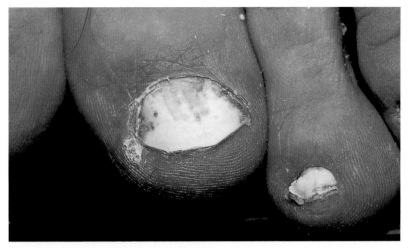

Figure 325. White superficial onychomycosis. The nail surface is white, keratotic, and powdery in white superficial onychomycosis. The organism is usually *Trichophyton mentagrophytes*.

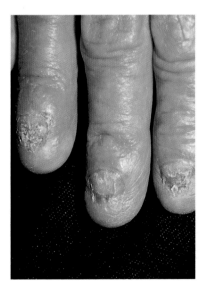

Figure 326. Chronic mucocutaneous candidiasis is a primary immune deficiency presenting as an inability to clear fungal infections and consequently as persisting and recurring infections of the nails, paronychial area, skin, and mucosa with yeasts, mostly *Candida albicans*. Various associations have included endocrinopathies, thymoma, interstitial keratitis, and susceptibility to other infectious agents. Both autosomal dominant and autosomal recessive inherited forms occur. Total nail destruction commonly occurs as shown here.

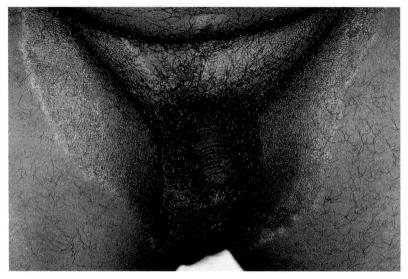

Figure 327. Tinea cruris, male.   Red, scaly plaques radiating out from the inguinal fold onto the inner thigh are characteristic of tinea cruris. The border is usually scaly, raised and KOH positive. Itching may vary from absent to severe.

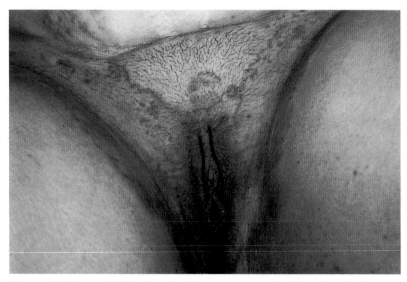

Figure 328. Tinea cruris, female.   Rarely, a woman may develop a dermatophyte infection of the groin.

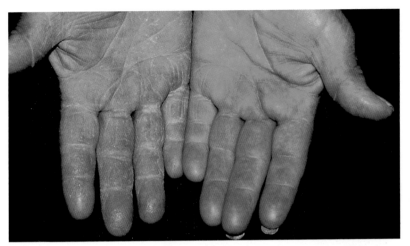

Figure 329. Two foot, one hand disease.　Chronic scaling of both feet and the dominant hand secondary to a fungal infection occurs in two foot, one hand disease. Unilateral onychomycosis may be present in chronic cases. Often the patient thinks the scaling is only caused by dry skin or physical trauma. Note the diffuse scale of the right hand without inflammation.

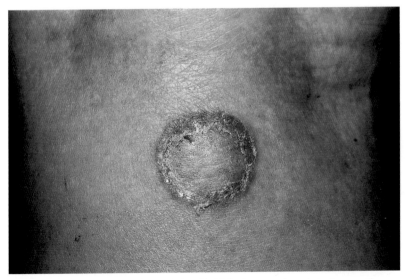

Figure 330. Tinea corporis, 'ringworm'.　Multiple, large, red, scaly lesions on the body, often with an active border, are characteristic. Nummular eczema, in contrast, usually shows uniform inflammation, scale, and/or crust throughout (see **Figure 255**).

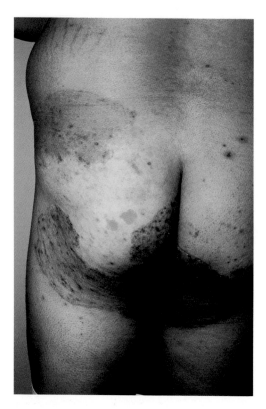

Figure 331. Tinea corporis. Multiple large plaques emanate from the folds onto the buttocks and trunk. Note the active border and the irregular, serpiginous margin. Small erythematous papules amidst the lesions are typical and represent fungal folliculitis.

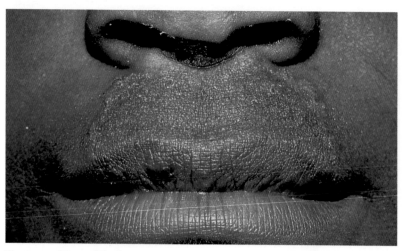

Figure 332. Tinea of the face.

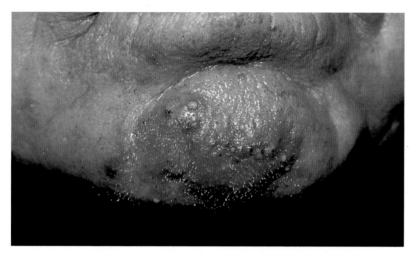

Figure 333. Tinea barbae. Fungal infection occasionally affects the beard area as annular, red, scaly rings, or as aggregated follicular pustules as shown here.

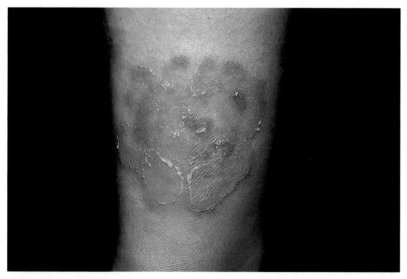

Figure 334. Majocchi's granuloma represents dermatophyte infection of dermal and/or subcutaneous tissue. The typical organism is *Trichophyton rubrum,* although other *Trychophyton* and *Microsporum* species may be found. Clinically, one sees a papulopustular perifollicular eruption on one leg of a woman who shaves. It is often mistaken for a bacterial folliculitis.

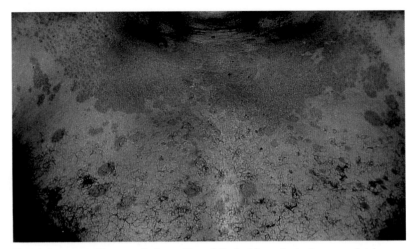

Figures 335–338. Tinea versicolor. Tinea (pityriasis) versicolor is a superficial infection of the stratum corneum by the lipophilic fungus of the *Malassezia* species. The most common predisposing factor is excessive sweating, but others include application of oils, systemic steroids, and, rarely, adrenocorticalism. Hyperpigmented (**Figure 335**, top) or hypopigmented (**Figure 336**, bottom) patches on the upper back of a young adult with a slight scale when scraped (**Figure 337**, on page 171) are characteristic. The chest and neck may also be affected. Often the most bothersome aspect for the patient is the lesion's inability to tan. A potassium hydroxide preparation of the scale (**Figure 338**, on page 171) shows short hyphae and budding cells ('spaghetti and meatballs').

Figures 336. Tinea versicolor, hypopigmented lesion. Both the infection and inflammation of tinea versicolor can disturb the pigmentary layer of the skin. Hyperpigmented and hypopigmented lesions may result.

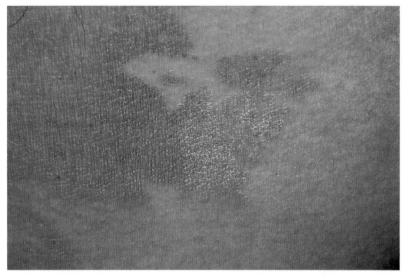

Figure 337. Tinea versicolor.   Note the slight scale when scraped.

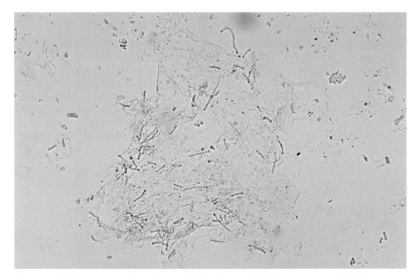

Figure 338. Tinea versicolor.   'Spaghetti and meatballs' appearance of KOH preparation of scale. (Courtesy Terence C O'Grady, MD.)

DEEP FUNGAL AND TROPICAL INFECTIONS

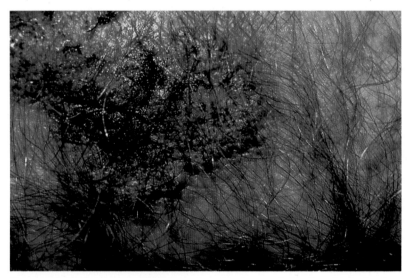

Figure 339. North American blastomycosis.   Blastomycosis is a fungal infection by *Blastomyces dermatitidis*. It is endemic to the Ohio and Mississippi river basins. It is a round yeast (diameter 8–15 µm) with broad-based budding and doubly refractile walls. Most cases of blastomycosis begin as a primary pulmonary infection after inhalation of the organism. Clinically, one sees solitary or multiple lesions that begin as papulonodules and slowly enlarge to form verrucous, vegetating plaques, often with central clearing. Within these lesions, pustules, exudates, and crust may form. Diagnosis is usually made by skin biopsy from which the organisms may be identified and cultured.

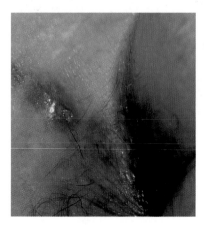

Figure 340. Coccidiomycosis is an infection caused by *Coccidioides immitis* and is indigenous to the southwestern USA, Mexico, and Central and South America. About half of patients with systemic infection develop cutaneous lesions. Rarely, patients may develop primary cutaneous coccidiomycosis. In either case, lesions may present as multiple papulopustules, papulonodules, granulomatous papules or plaques, ulcers (as shown here), and subcutaneous abscess.

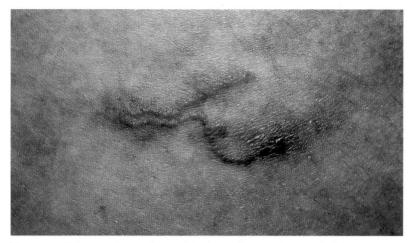

Figure 341. Cutaneous larva migrans (also known as creeping eruption) is a characteristic eruption that is caused by penetration and migration in the skin of nematode larvae. In the USA, *Acnylostoma caninum* or *A. brasiliensis* (dog or cat hookworm) is common. The patient usually acquires the infection from wet sand or dirt contaminated with animal feces. Clinically, one sees a red, pruritic linear eruption on the foot, back, or thigh. This 20-year-old woman developed this lesion on her left hip after spending time in Mexico.

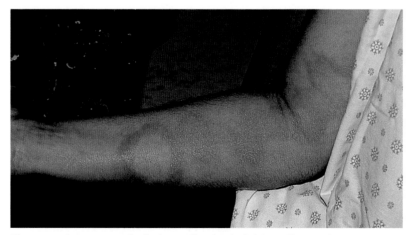

Figure 342. Leprosy, annular lesion. The classic division of leprosy is into a tuberculoid (paucibacillary, few organisms, high resistance) and a lepromatous (multibacillary, many organisms, low resistance) type with borderline between the two. The typical lesion in the tuberculoid type is a large annular erythematous plaque with an involuting, hypopigmented, anesthetic center. Nerve enlargement (e.g. greater auricular, superficial peroneal) with muscle atrophy may occur.

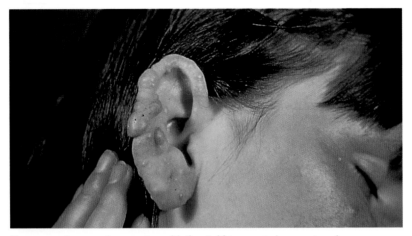

Figure 343. Leprosy, lepromatous, histiocytoid type. In lepromatous leprosy, nodular infiltration of the face, ears, and elsewhere may occur. The eyebrows may be progressively lost. Note the nodular infiltration of the ear in this teenage Peruvian girl. (Courtesy of James Steger, MD.)

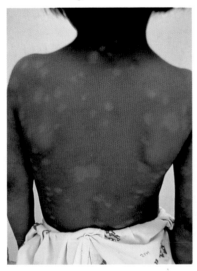

Figure 344. Leprosy, borderline tuberculoid. Note the multiple, hypopigmented lesions. (Courtesy of James Steger, MD.)

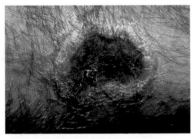

Figure 345. Leishmaniasis, ulcer. An inflammatory red–brown papulonodule develops initially at the site of a bite by the sand fly, usually on the face, neck, or arms. The incubation period is usually several months but may be from a few days to over a year. The lesion enlarges to a crusted nodule. The crust may then fall off, leaving a large ulcer (as shown here on the arm) that later heals with a scar.

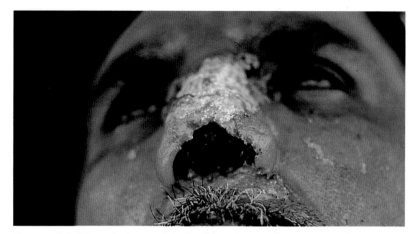

Figure 346. Leishmaniasis, nasal destruction. In a small percentage of cases, infection by *Leishmania brasiliensis* may spread to the nasopharyngeal mucosa, causing significant destruction. (Courtesy of James Steger, MD.)

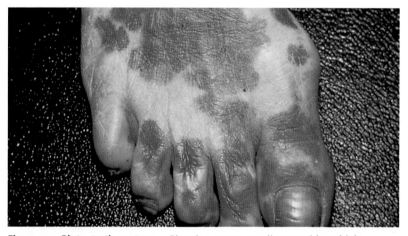

Figure 347. Pinta, tertiary stage. Pinta is a cutaneous disease with multiple stages caused by the non-venereal spirochete *Treponema carateum*. It is the most benign of the spirochetal diseases, causing primarily skin changes. Pinta has mostly disappeared worldwide except for some areas of Brazil. One case was recently described in Austria, imported possibly from Cuba. In the primary stage of pinta, a minute macule or papule develops at the site of inoculation and spreads to form a large (10–12.5 cm), poorly defined, erythematous infiltrated plaque. In the secondary stage, pintids form that are red, violaceous, blue, brown, gray, or black papulosquamous plaques. They may fade and relapse, forming polycyclic lesions. In the tertiary or late dyschromic stage of pinta, which occurs months to a decade after the pintids, depigmented patches develop as shown here. (Courtesy of James Steger, MD.)

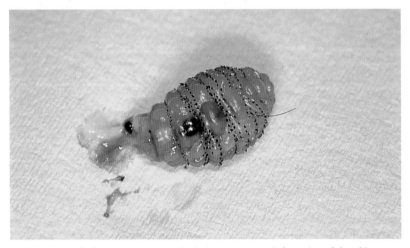

Figure 348. Myiasis. Cutaneous myiasis is a temporary infestation of the skin with fly larvae order Diptera, e.g. *Dermatobia hominis*, and is a common disease endemic in tropical zones. The adult female lays eggs on the ground that hatch to first-stage larvae. They then penetrate the skin of a warm-blooded animal (e.g. a human lying on the ground or sand) and mature to adult larvae. The larvae then fall to the ground and turn into flies.

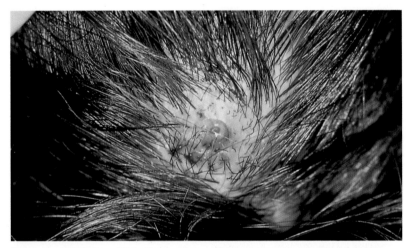

Figure 349. Myiasis. Clinically, one sees multiple, scattered red, papulonodules much like furuncles that may drain a serosanguinous fluid (**Figure 349**, bottom). (Courtesy of Stacy Smith, MD.)

SEXUALLY TRANSMITTED AND OTHER GENITAL DISEASES

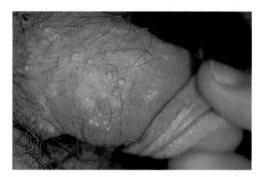

Figure 350. Molluscum contagiosum. Lesions of molluscum on the lower abdomen and groin of adults are often transmitted during sexual contact. In contrast, genital lesions in children in most cases are innocently obtained. (See also **Figure 91**.)

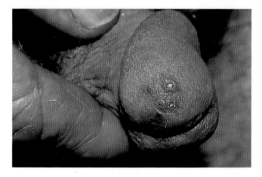

Figure 351. Herpes genitalis, male. Most cases of herpes of the genitalia are caused by HSV-2, but some are caused by HSV-1. The classic appearance of grouped vesicles on an erythematous base is usually not seen. Instead, localized pain, erosions, or erythema may be the only features. Primary infection can be painful, and individual outbreaks usually last from several days to a week. Recurrent episodes are often of shorter duration. Over time, recurrences tend to be less frequent. Stressful events of at least 7 days' duration significantly predict recurrences. Asymptomatic shedding is an important factor in spread of the disease.

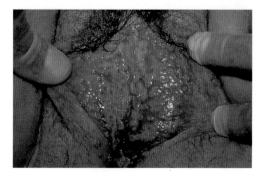

Figure 352. Herpes genitalis, female. (Courtesy of Michael O Murphy, MD.)

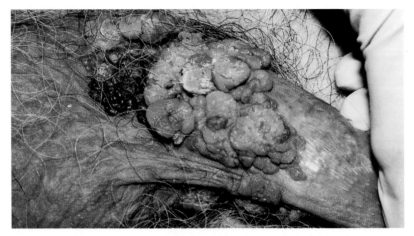

Figure 353. Condyloma acuminata, penis. The term condyloma (knuckle) acuminata (pointed) was originally coined to describe the often pointed or exuberant morphology of this condition in contrast to the syphilitic lesions of condyloma lata. The cutaneous lesions are caused by infection by the human papilloma virus (HPV). This is the most common sexually transmitted disease. HPV infection is associated with dysplasia or frank malignancy of the uterine cervix in women. The HPV types can be separated into low (6, 11), intermediate (31, 33, 35), and high risk (16, 18). The term bowenoid papulosis is used when the histologic picture of a lesion resembles Bowen's diseases. Clinically, one sees smooth or papillomatous papules or nodules on the penis, scrotum, perianally, and on the skin of the groin in men. In women, lesions may occur on the vulva, labia, intravaginally, or on the cervix. Lesions may be flesh-colored, tan, or brown. All patients with genital lesions should have a perianal exam to exclude perianal involvement.

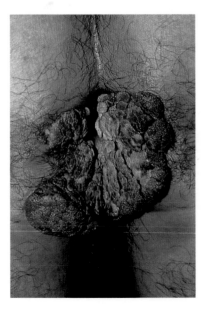

Figure 354. Condyloma acuminata, perianal. The viral particles causing perianal condyloma may have originated from warts elsewhere on the body and been transmitted via the patient's own hands, or they may have been contracted during anal sex. (See also **Figure 93**.)

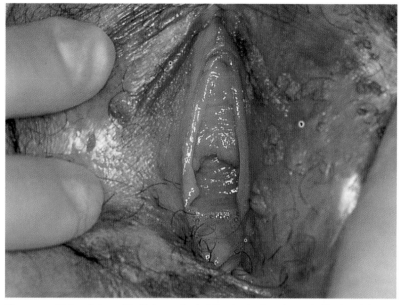

Figure 355. Vulvar intraepithelial neoplasia III. In the female genitalia, condyloma acuminata and bowenoid papulosis are sometimes grouped under the term vulvar intraepithelial neoplasia, and the atypia graded from I to III. Erythematous or pigmented, smooth or papillomatous papules, sometimes coalescent into nodules, are characteristic. Human papilloma virus, especially type 16, has been found in a significant percentage of lesions, and thus the patient should be monitored for atypia of the uterine cervix. (Courtesy of Paul Koonings, MD.)

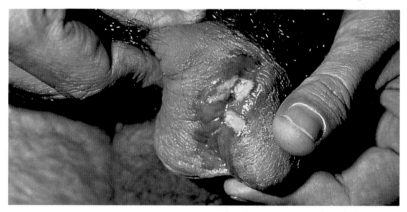

Figure 356. Primary syphilis, chancre. Syphilis is caused by *Treponema pallidum*. In primary syphilis, solitary or multiple, painless ulcers or erosions called chancres occur. They tend to remain superficial but may become indurated. In women, the chancres may occur in the vagina or on the cervix and go unnoticed. Chancres may occur at other sites of inoculation (e.g. the anus in a homosexual man, the mouth after oral sex). (Courtesy of Department of Dermatology, University of California, San Diego.)

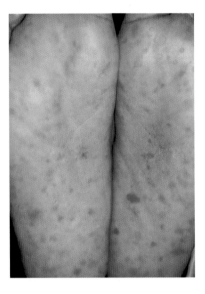

Figure 357. Secondary syphilis, papulosquamous lesions, soles. Approximately 6 weeks after the chancre, malaise, headache, fever, lymphadenopathy, and a mucocutaneous eruption develop. A widespread papulosquamous eruption of ham-to-copper-hued lesions with a predilection for the palms and soles is characteristic. Scale, when present, tends to be located at the periphery. Necrotic or nodular forms occur. (Courtesy of Theodore Sebastien, MD.)

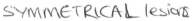

SYMMETRICAL lesions

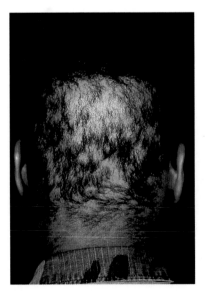

Figure 358. Secondary syphilis, moth-eaten alopecia. Patchy, 'moth-eaten' alopecia affects the scalp, eyebrows, eyelashes, and beard. (Courtesy of Stacy Smith, MD.)

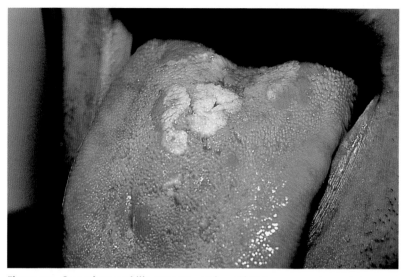

Figure 359. Secondary syphilis, mucous patch. Whitish-gray papules and plaques may occur on the tongue, or other mucous membrane surfaces.

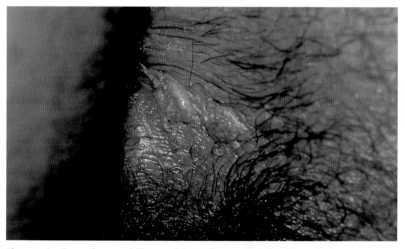

Figure 360. Secondary syphilis, condyloma lata, perianal. These lesions are teeming with *Treponema pallidum*.

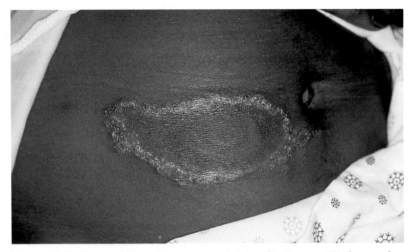

Figure 361. Tertiary syphilis. The cutaneous lesions of tertiary syphilis (gummas) are often polycyclic or serpiginous with central ulceration or clearing. These granulomatous lesions are usually painless but may be locally destructive. Gummatous lesions may develop internally as well. (Courtesy of Department of Dermatology, University of California, San Diego.)

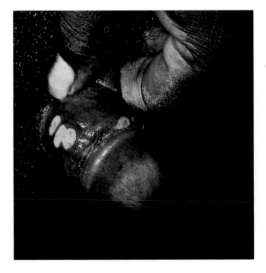

Figure 362. Chancroid is a common cause of genital ulcers worldwide. The Gram-negative bacillus *Haemophilus ducreyi* has a 'school of fish' appearance on smear. Clinically, the lesions tend to be painful and foul smelling. (Courtesy of Michael O Murphy, MD.)

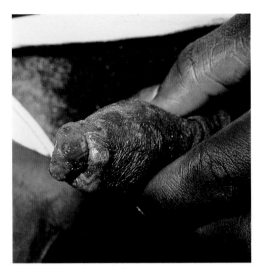

Figure 363. Granuloma inguinale is an indolent, progressive, ulcerative, and granulomatous disease of the genitalia caused by the Gram-negative bacterium *Calymmatobacterium granulomatis*. Giemsa or Wright's stain of a tissue smear or skin biopsy specimen shows intracytoplasmic inclusion bodies (Donovan bodies) within histiocytes. The ulcer tends to be beefy yet asymptomatic with exuberant granulation tissue.

One other infectious agent classically causes a genital erosion: *Chlamydia trachomatis* causes lymphogranuloma venerium. The genital lesion typically is a small erosion that goes unnoticed. One to two weeks later, firm lymphadenopathy develops. The classic 'groove' sign is created by enlarged inguinal and femoral nodes separated by Poupart's ligament.

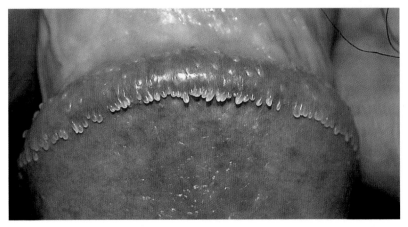

Figure 364. Pearly penile papules.   Two or three rows of uniform, flesh-colored papules running circumferentially about the corona are characteristic. Onset is typically noted in the 20s and 30s. These papules may be mistaken for warts but are not infectious.

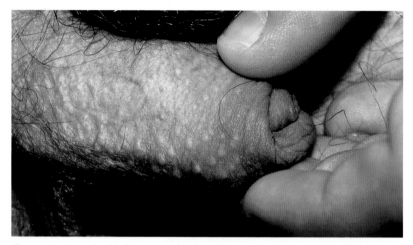

Figure 365. Tyson's glands, or prominent sebaceous glands, are commonly seen along the shaft of the penis. They are ectopic sebaceous glands and appear unassociated with the hair follicle. Knowledge of their existence helps prevent confusion with condyloma. They appear as 1–2 mm uniform papules at the base of hairs and are seen in about one third of men. They may number more than 100 and are more common on the ventral surface.

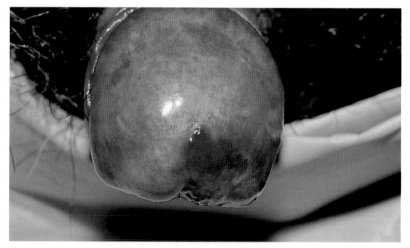

Figure 366. Zoon's balanitis, also known as balanitis plasmocellularis, is an uncommon, benign, idiopathic inflammatory condition of older, uncircumcised men. A moist, shiny, erythematous, well-demarcated plaque on the glans penis in an older uncircumcised male is characteristic.

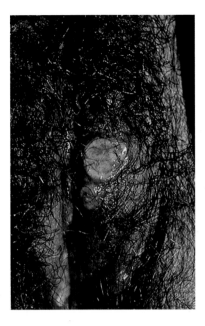

Figure 367. Behçet's disease, vulva.
Behçet's syndrome is an inflammatory condition whose most characteristic features are recurrent oral and genital ulcerations. Ocular, arthritic, neurological, vascular, GI, and pulmonary lesions may occur as well. The oral ulcerations resemble aphthosis. The genital ulcerations may affect the labia, vaginal introitus, or scrotum. Deep, tender nodules of the shins resembling erythema nodosum are not uncommon. Scattered inflammatory, acneiform papules and pustules may be seen. Uncommon cutaneous manifestations include polyarteritis nodosa, Sweet's syndrome-like lesions, pyoderma gangrenosum-like lesions, erythema multiforme-like lesions, infiltrated erythema, palpable purpura, hemorrhagic bulla, superficial migratory thrombophlebitis, extragenital ulcerations, thrombophlebitis, and pathergy. Nail fold capillary abnormalities are present in most patients with Behçet's disease.

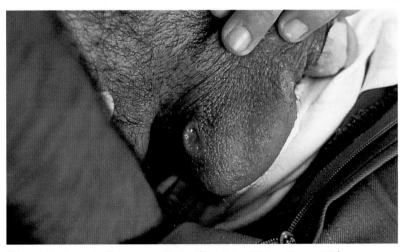

Figure 368. Behçet's disease, scrotum.   (Courtesy of Erkan Alpsoy, MD.)

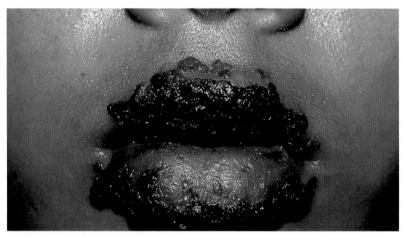

Figure 369. Herpes labialis, primary.   This crusting, vesicular, primary herpes simplex virus (HSV) infection of the lips and/or the oropharynx is most common in children. Fever and lymphadenopathy may occur. HSV-1 is the predominant pathogen.

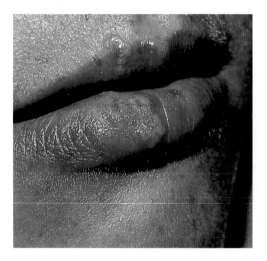

Figure 370. Herpes labialis, recurrent.   Pain or tingling followed by grouped vesicles on an erythematous base on the lip, typically centered on the vermilion border but also on nearby sites, is characteristic of this recurrent infection by HSV. Triggering factors for herpes labialis include dental work, fever, UV radiation, local trauma, mental stress, or menstruation.

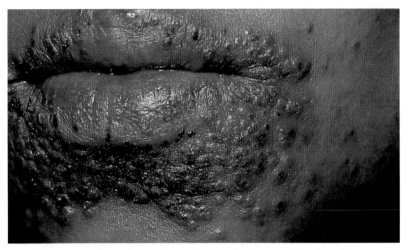

Figure 371. Eczema herpeticum refers to herpes simplex superinfection of eczematous skin. Patients with atopic dermatitis are particularly prone to this condition. It is signaled by the acute eruption of diffuse vesicles that quickly rupture leaving erosions and crusting. (See also **Figures 49** and **50**.)

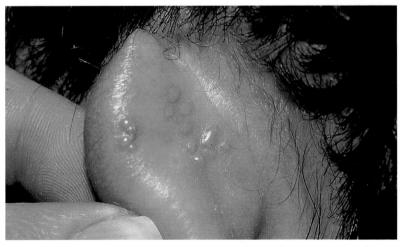

Figure 372. Herpes simplex, pustular.   After several days, the clear vesicles of herpes become pustules.

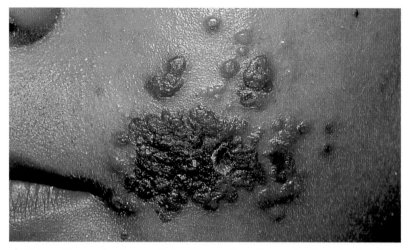

Figure 373. Herpes simplex, crusted. The crusting of herpes is often mistaken for impetigo, especially in children. Always look for intact vesicles and pustules among the crust. Bacterial and viral cultures are invaluable.

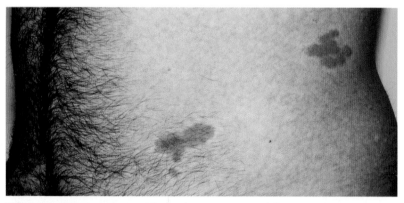

Figure 374. Herpes zoster, or shingles, is an acute vesiculobullous eruption caused by reactivation of the varicella zoster virus. (Zoster means girdle and derives from the dermatomal distribution of the rash.) Varicella zoster virus (VZV) causes both chickenpox and herpes zoster. After a bout of chickenpox, the VZV remains latent in nerve ganglion cells, typically sensory cells, for years. Reactivation of the virus occurs as the immune system surveillance wanes, typically in older age. The sexes are equally affected, and the incidence increases with age. Children only rarely develop zoster. Groups of vesicles, each on an erythematous base scattered within a dermatome, are characteristic. The trunk and face are most commonly affected. The lesions stop at the midline. Intense pain may incapacitate the patient. A few lesions may be found outside the dermatome; however, generalization of the zoster may occur, especially in those with decreased cellular immunity. Post-herpetic neuralgia (defined as pain beyond 4 weeks) is a potentially debilitating sequela. The risk of it developing increases significantly after the age of 60 years.

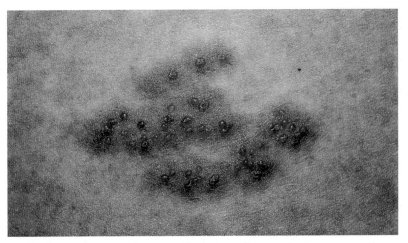

Figure 375. Herpes zoster, close up. The lesions of herpes simplex may occur in scattered islands, as shown here, or they may be confluent. Early in the course of the disease, a single island of grouped vesicles may present and be hard to distinguish from herpes simplex.

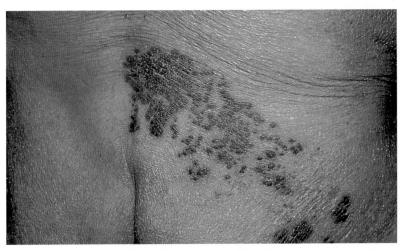

Figure 376. Herpes zoster, hemorrhagic. The vesicles of herpes zoster may at times be hemorrhagic.

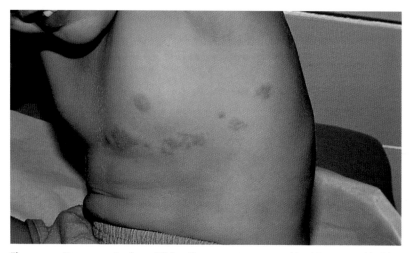

Figure 377. Herpes zoster in a child.   Herpes zoster occurred in this 3-year-old girl. She had chickenpox at 18 months. The varicella zoster virus causes both conditions. Spontaneous resolution can be expected.

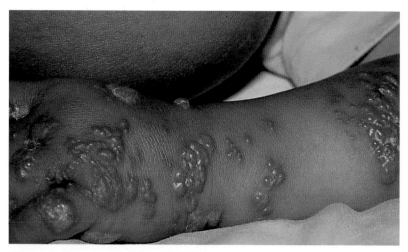

Figure 378. Herpes zoster in immunocompromised host.   Shingles preferentially affects those with decreased cellular immunity, e.g. elderly people, HIV-positive patients, and those with hematologic malignancy. This 3-year-old with leukemia developed shingles on the left arm.

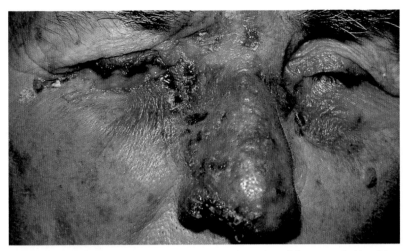

Figure 379. Ophthalmologic zoster. Vesicles and crusting of the top and side of the nose in herpes zoster implies involvement of the nasociliary branch of the trigeminal nerve and eye involvement. Ocular scarring and loss of vision may occur.

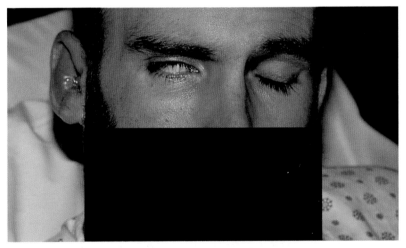

Figure 380. Ramsay–Hunt syndrome. Herpes zoster of the geniculate ganglion, resulting in vesicles of the ear (shown here) and tympanic membrane, occurs in Ramsay–Hunt syndrome. Both the 7th and 8th cranial nerve functions may be affected. Patients may have tinnitus, deafness, nausea, vomiting, nystagmus, facial hemiplegia, and partial loss of taste. The patient shown is trying to close both eyes.

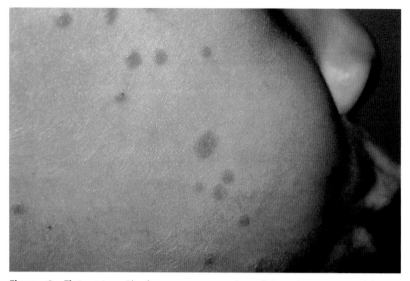

Figure 381. Flat warts.   Also known as verruca plana, flat warts present as pink, flesh-colored or tan, flat-topped, slightly elevated papules common on the forehead, face, and dorsa of the hands and legs. The lesions are typically caused by HPV 3. Flat warts on the face may take on a tan color and resemble multiple nevi.

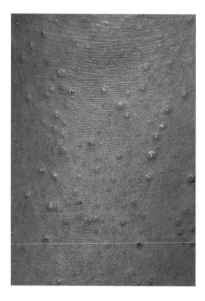

Figure 382. Flat warts, legs. The shaved legs of teenage women are commonly affected by flat warts. The razor seems to spread the infection. Tiny papules around many of the hairs are seen.

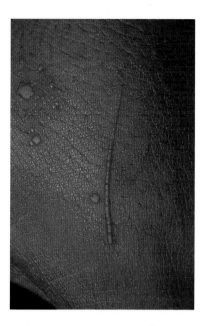

Figure 383. Flat warts, Köbnerization. Köbnerization refers to the development of a disease at the site of epidermal injury. Here scratching has caused the warts to form in a line.

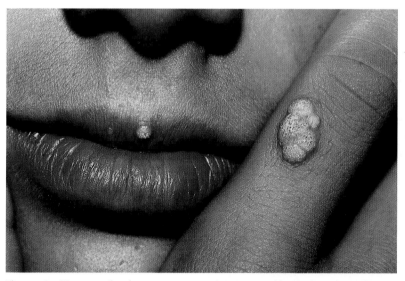

Figure 384. Verruca vulgaris, or common warts, are caused by the human papilloma virus. Warts come in many shapes and sizes. Solitary or multiple hyperkeratotic or verrucous papules on the hands or fingers of a child or adolescent are characteristic. The normal skin lines are obscured. Warts on the hands are very common and may affect all ages but with the preponderance from age 5–25 years.

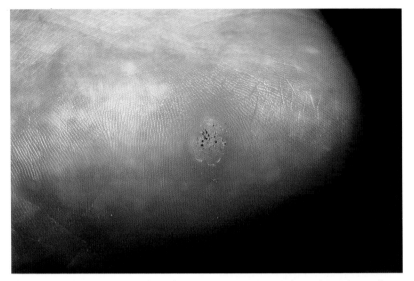

Figure 385. Plantar wart.   A hyperkeratotic, verrucous papule or plaque beneath a pressure point on the sole of the foot is characteristic. Paring reveals black dots as shown here, which represent thrombosed capillaries. HPV types 1 (myrmecia), 2 (mosaic), and 4 are most common. Because plantar warts are driven into the skin by the pressure of walking or standing, they are usually the most resistant to treatment.

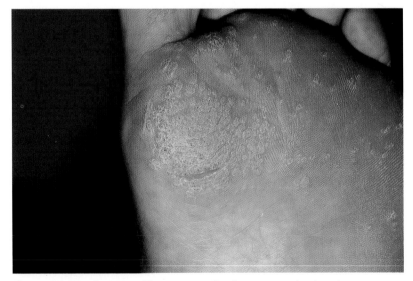

Figure 386. Mosaic warts.   The term mosaic refers to warts that have become confluent, forming a hyperkeratotic plaque. Mosaic warts most commonly occur on the soles.

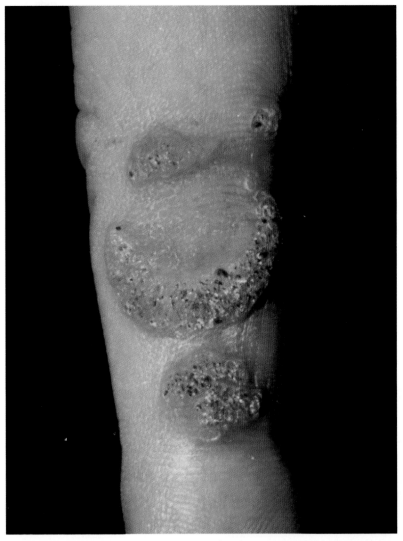

Figure 387. Donut wart. It is not uncommon for warts to recur at the edges of cryotherapy, creating the shape of a donut. (The middle lesion pictured here perhaps resembles more a crescent roll.)

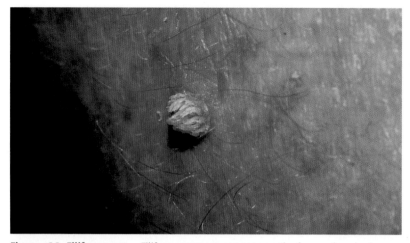

Figure 388. Filiform wart. Filiform warts are common on the face and neck of adults. Their shape is reminiscent of a horse's tail.

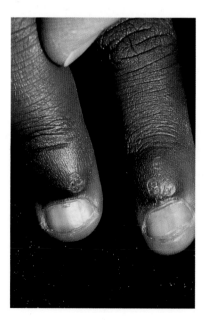

Figure 389. Verruca, periungual. Warts about the nails are common in children. Their presence may depress the matrix, causing a groove in the nail. Care must be taken not to damage the matrix when treating such verrucae, or else permanent damage to the nail may result.

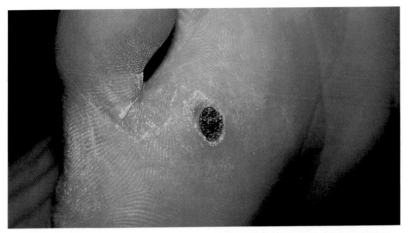

Figure 390. Regressing plantar wart. Spontaneous blackening of a plantar wart is a sign of imminent regression. It is as if the immune system suddenly did not like the wart and decided to get rid of it. Erythema and pruritus may precede this color change. After turning black, the wart just peels and falls off.

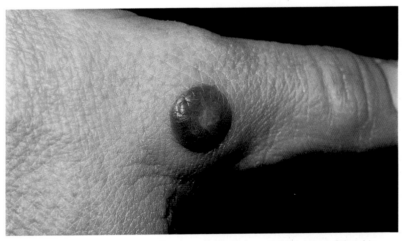

Figure 391. Orf, also known as ecthyma contagiosa, is a viral infection of the skin usually acquired from a goat or sheep. It is usually an occupational hazard seen in farmers, shepherds, veterinarians, and abattoir workers. The orf virus belongs to the parapox subgroup of the pox viruses. A solitary papulonodule develops at the site of inoculation. Fever, lymphadenopathy, and erythema multiforme may accompany the lesion.

See also neonatal herpes (**Figure 31**), molluscum contagiosum (**Figure 91**), measles (**Figure 117**), roseola (**Figure 121**), chickenpox (**Figure 133**), and hand, foot, and mouth disease (**Figure 135**).

INFESTATIONS AND BITES

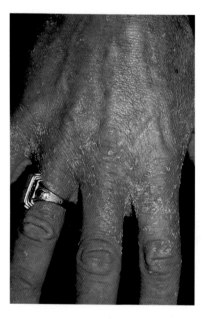

Figure 392. Scabies, hand. Scabies represents an infestation of the skin by the mite *Sarcoptes scabiei var hominis*. The organism creates tunnels (burrows) in the keratin layer of the skin, laying eggs, and leaving feces (scybala). These burrows are most visible on the inner wrists, sides of the feet, and web spaces of the fingers. They appear as linear, thread-like burrows often with a black dot at one end (the mite). Over time, lichenification, excoriations, scabetic nodules and secondary bacterial infection may develop. This diagnosis may be very difficult to make in the patient who scratches away the burrows. Close-up examination of the scaly lesions in this patient shows many of them to be linear. The patient experiences intense itching because they are allergic to the mite, its eggs and feces. Often, the itching is the most severe at night, but this is partly because the patient is not distracted by their duties of the day. All patients whose predominant complaint is itching should have their web spaces, wrists, and feet examined.

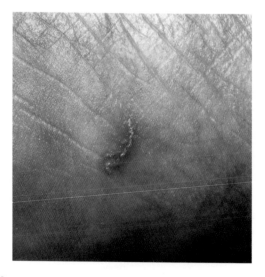

Figure 393. Scabies, burrow. The sides of the feet are excellent places to find burrows. Note the linear, thread-like, serpiginous scale. Occasionally, the patient with scabies will complain only of a hand dermatitis or a penile eruption. The patient should fully disrobe to allow examination of the axilla, trunk, waist, and groin.

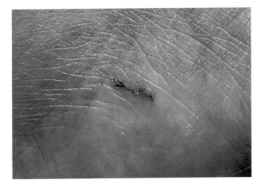

Figure 394. Scabies, burrow, ink test. The ink test is performed by rubbing the skin with black ink and then wiping it off. If burrows are present, the ink will run down into them and remain. Note the V-shaped ending of this burrow at 10 o'clock. This is where the skin is shedding the last remnants of that portion of the burrow. The end pointing to 4 o'clock is where the scabies mite is still actively burrowing.

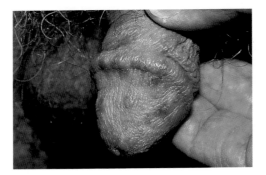

Figure 395. Scabies, nodular lesions, penis. The penis is almost always affected in some fashion in men with scabies. Nodular lesions, as shown here, often develop.

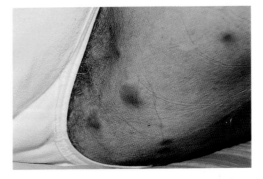

Figure 396. Scabies, nodular lesions, thigh. Multiple red–brown papulonodules may develop in the patient who has had scabies for several months. The inner thigh is affected in this patient.

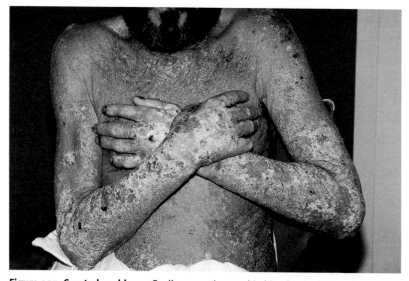

Figure 397. Crusted scabies.   Scaling, crusting, and itching beginning on the hands, feet, and groin and progressing to cover the entire body are characteristic. Thousands of mites have populated the skin, in contrast to conventional scabies in which the number is thought to be less than 20. Patients usually have neurological disease (e.g. Down's syndrome, mental retardation) or immunosuppression (e.g. AIDS, hematologic malignancy).

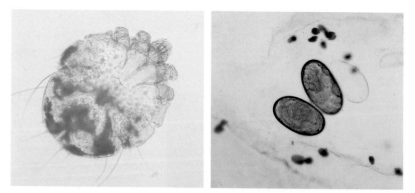

Figure 398. Scabies, microscopic examination.   Affected skin is scraped with a blade moistened with mineral oil. The resultant mix is applied to a slide, covered with a cover-slip and examined microscopically. The presence of even a single mite (left), egg, or scybala (right) is diagnostic. (Courtesy of Morse, Moreland and Holmes, *Atlas of Sexually Transmitted Diseases and AIDS*, Mosby-Wolfe, 1996.)

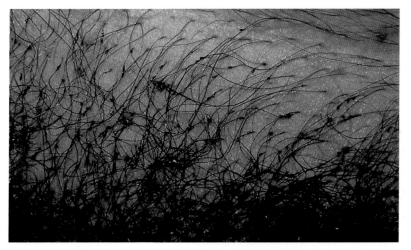

Figure 399. Pediculosis pubis, groin.   Pubic, head, and body lice are blood-sucking and host-specific for humans. The technical name for pubic lice is *Phthirus pubis*. Pruritus of the groin is often the only symptom of pediculosis pubis. Inspection of the area shows small, ovoid nits (eggs) attached firmly to the hair and pointing away from the skin. Closer inspection will show crab-like organisms hanging to the base of adjacent hairs. This disease is spread by close physical (e.g. sexual) contact.

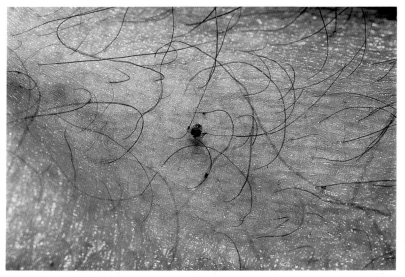

Figure 400. Pediculosis pubis, abdomen.   The organisms may spread upward to the abdomen and chest as shown here.

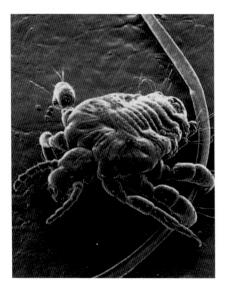

Figure 401. Pediculosis pubis.
The pubic louse is shown here.
(Courtesy of Morse, Moreland and
Holmes, *Atlas of Sexually
Transmitted Diseases and AIDS*,
Mosby-Wolfe, 1996.)

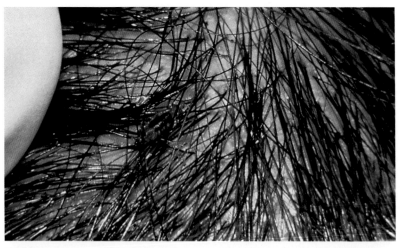

Figure 402. Pediculosis capitis, adult. Lice suck the patient's blood and leave
behind digestive material and feces. Intense pruritus results. Secondary infection and
alopecia from scratching may occur. Head and body lice are caused by distinct
variants of *Pediculus humanus*.

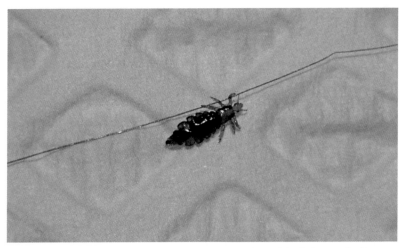

Figure 403. Pediculosis capitis, louse. Close inspection of the hair reveals the wingless louse. Note that the head and body louse have longer, more slender bodies than the pubic louse, which is more crab-like.

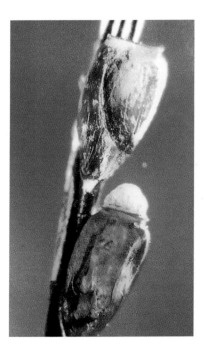

Figure 404. Pediculosis capitis, nit. The egg (nit) is shown firmly cemented to the hair shaft. (Courtesy of Morse, Moreland and Holmes, *Atlas of Sexually Transmitted Diseases and AIDS*, Mosby-Wolfe, 1996.)

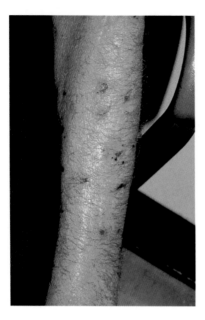

Figure 405. Pediculosis corporis.
Excoriations, crusting and urticarial papules may be seen in pediculosis corporis. The lice live on the clothes and descend onto the skin to feed. Any part of the skin covered by clothes may be affected. Usually it is the homeless or other indigent patients who do not routinely wash their clothes that are affected.

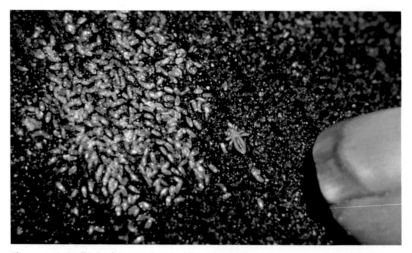

Figure 406. Pediculosis corporis, clothing plus louse. Inspection of the clothing allows for diagnosis.

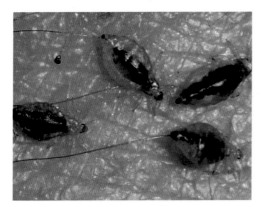

Figure 407. Pediculosis corporis, louse. (Courtesy of Peters and Gilles, *Color Atlas of Tropical Medicine and Parasitology*, 4th edn, Mosby-Wolfe, 1995 and Dr med H Lieske.)

Analysis of the specimens sent to us on February 26, 1993 revealed the following:

Dry scalp _____

Lice _____

Mites _____

Ants _____

Slugs _____

Other _____

Your diligence in obtaining and mailing these "bugs" for our examination is appreciated.

Sincerely,

Mr. White
Dermatology Department

Figure 408. Delusions of parasitosis is a rare psychiatric disorder in which patients falsely believe that their skin is infested with parasites. Even though it is a psychiatric disorder, these patients usually present to a dermatologist because they are convinced that they have a dermatological problem. Patients with delusions of parasitosis generally reject psychiatric referral. The patient may go in and out of a delusional state. (A delusion is an idea that the patient holds to firmly and cannot in any way be convinced of otherwise. A patient who will honestly consider the possibility that they do not have bugs is not strictly delusional.) The condition may be primary or secondary to a variety of disorders, including drug use (e.g. alcohol, cocaine, or amphetamines), organic brain dysfunction, or schizophrenia. A toxicology screen may be needed. The physician must always rule out true infestation, e.g. by scabies, pediculosis, the rat mite, bird mite, etc. This author once saw an elderly woman who complained of ants crawling on her skin. When asked to bring them in, she did! Fumigating the house cured the problem. Patients may be encouraged to bring in specimens for microscopic examination. This patient even provided a form to fill out!

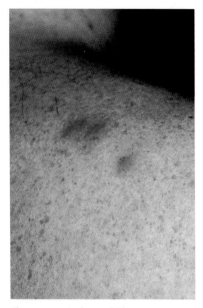

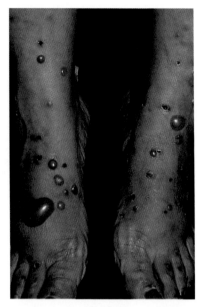

Figure 409. Arthropod bite. Spiders, mosquitoes, or other arthropods may bite almost any part of the body. The individual papules are red, grouped, and intensely itchy. The bug whose bites are shown here had breakfast, lunch, and dinner!

Figure 410. Flea bite, bullae. Flea bites occur about the ankles because these tiny brown insects can jump no higher than 2 feet (60 cm). Vesicles and bullae may occur. Because the host's immune response is important in pathogenesis, only one member of the family may be affected. (See also **Figure 102.**)

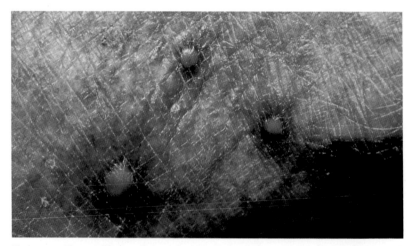

Figure 411. Fire ant bites. Intense burning and pain are associated with the bites of fire ants. A wheal is followed by a vesicle, which finally forms a pustule as shown here. This woman had stepped on a group of ants 7 days before presenting.

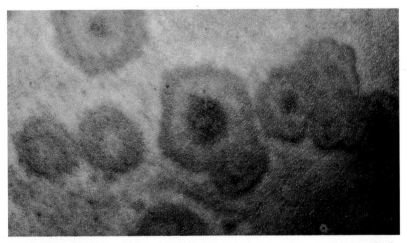

Figure 412. Erythema multiforme, target lesion. Classic erythema multiforme (EM) is an inflammatory response often associated with herpes virus infection that creates a target lesion in the skin. These target lesions (concentric rings of different shades of red) may have a dusky, necrotic, or bullous center. The dorsum of the hand is one of the most commonly affected sites. Some use the term EM broadly to describe any diffuse urticarial red rash, whereas others require the presence of target lesions for the condition to qualify as EM.

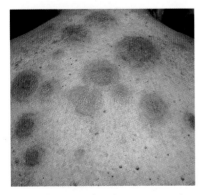

Figure 413. Sweet's syndrome.
Also known as acute febrile neutrophilic dermatosis, Sweet's syndrome is an acute eruption that occurs in response to a variety of antigens and is characterized by a neutrophilic infiltrate in the skin. A preceding respiratory infection is perhaps the most characteristic precipitant, but others include other infections (e.g. tonsillitis, vulvovaginal infections, HIV, coccidiomycosis, *Chlamydia trachomatis*), inflammatory diseases (e.g. inflammatory bowel disease, SLE, RA, Sjögren's syndrome), solid carcinomas (e.g. breast, stomach, prostate, colon), and hemoproliferative diseases (e.g. leukemia, myelodysplasia, lymphoma). It may present with fever, leukocytosis, and rapidly developing painful, red plaques on the upper back, arms, face, neck, or elsewhere. The abdomen, lower back, buttocks, and posterior thighs tend to be spared. The surface of these plaques may exhibit a mamillated appearance, pustules, pseudovesiculation, or crusting. Erythema nodosum-like lesions may occur on the legs and arms. (Courtesy of Michael O Murphy, MD.)

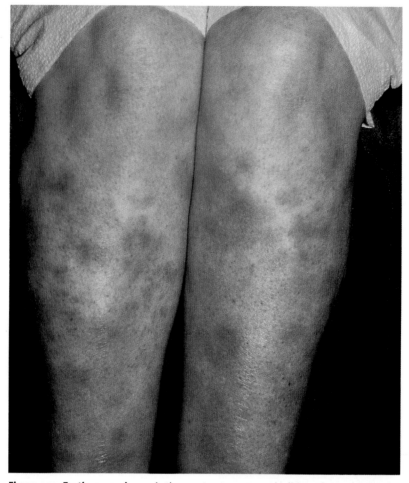

Figure 414. Erythema nodosum is the most common panniculitis and may develop in response to a wide variety of antigens. Precipitating factors include various infections (e.g. streptococcal, tuberculosis, coccidiomycosis (shown here), blastomycosis, histoplasmosis, *Yersinia* species, salmonella enteritis, *Chlamydia trachomatis*, milker's nodules, tularemia, or hepatitis B), drugs (e.g. birth control pills), pregnancy, ulcerative colitis, sarcoidosis, and rarely malignancy, e.g. lymphoma. Both Sweet's syndrome and cryoglobulinemia can cause lesions that resemble erythema nodosum. Work-up may include skin biopsy, complete blood count, urine analysis, antistreptolysin-O, throat culture, chest X-ray, liver enzymes, stool culture if diarrhea is present, and intradermal or serologic tests for deep fungi. Red, tender, deep-seated nodules scattered on both shins in an adult are characteristic. The disease usually runs its course over 3–6 weeks.

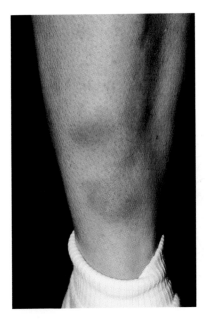

Figure 415. Villanova's disease.
A painless, erythematous nodule enlarging to a plaque on the lower aspect of one shin in a woman is characteristic of Villanova's disease, also called subacute nodular migratory panniculitis. The lesion may be chronic with slow expansion. The lesion is usually misdiagnosed as cellulitis, but the adept clinician will note its much slower onset and course, e.g. over weeks to months. Many consider this disease a variant of erythema nodosum and use the term erythema nodosum migrans.

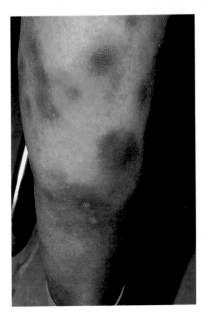

Figure 416. Nodular vasculitis.
Tender, red, deep-seated nodules, mainly on the calves, chiefly in women, are characteristic. Ulceration commonly occurs. A work-up to exclude tuberculosis should be done.
If tuberculosis is found, the term erythema induratum of Bazin is used.

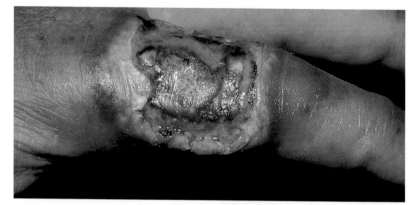

Figure 417. Neutrophilic dermatosis of the dorsal hands. Neutrophilic dermatosis (pustular vasculitis) of the dorsal hands is a recently described disorder, which may clinically and histologically resemble a localized variant of Sweet's syndrome. The patient presents with pustular or ulcerative plaques, nodules, and hemorrhagic bullae on the dorsal hands and/or fingers. When it ulcerates, the lesions may closely resemble pyoderma gangrenosum as shown here. A low grade fever may be present.

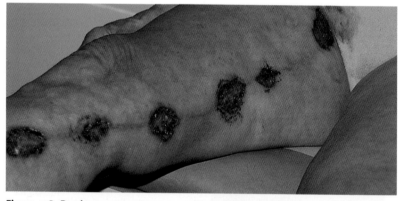

Figure 418. Pyoderma gangrenosum, multiple ulcers. Pyoderma gangrenosum is a non-infectious ulcerative disease classically associated with chronic inflammatory conditions such as ulcerative colitis, Crohn's disease, arthritis, chronic active hepatitis, and Takayasu's arteritis. In making the diagnosis, infection (e.g. deep fungal), malignancy (e.g. lymphoma), and vasculopathy (e.g. Wegener's granulomatosis, antiphospholipid syndrome) must be excluded. Beginning as a papule or pustule, the lesion breaks down to form an ulcer with an undermined, violaceous, jagged border. It commonly occurs on the legs but also elsewhere, and is often painful. Lesions may occur at sites of trauma (pathergy) as shown here after surgery. Work-up may include antinuculear antibodies (ANA), rheumatoid factor, hepatic and renal enzymes, complete blood count, rapid plasma reagin, serum protein electrophoresis, evaluation of the GI tract, and biopsy of the margin of the ulcer for histopathology and culture (e.g. bacterial, viral, fungal, atypical mycobacteria).

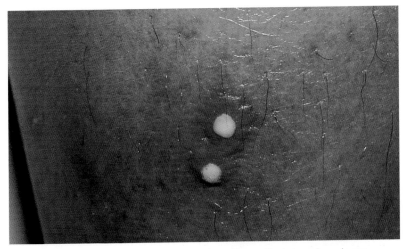

Figure 419. Pyoderma gangrenosum, pustule. The earliest sign of pyoderma gangrenosum may be a pustule.

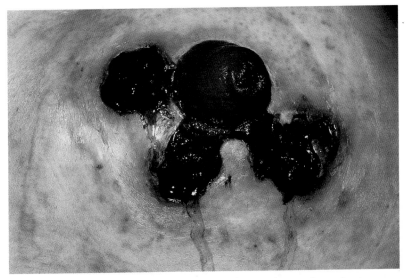

Figure 420. Pyoderma gangrenosum, periostomal. An ulcer or ulcers about an ostomy site may represent pyoderma gangrenosum. If Crohn's disease is the reason for the ostomy, involvement of the GI tract adjacent to the ostomy site should be considered.

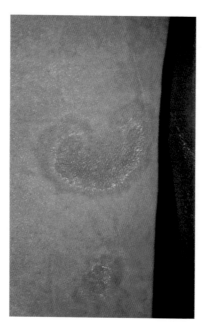

Figure 421. Erythema annulare centrificum is a distinct cutaneous eruption characterized by spreading annular lesions with a trailing scale. The morphology is distinct from that of tinea corporis, which classically has a scaly leading edge. Two clinical subtypes are recognized: a superficial gyrate erythema (scaly, pruritic) and a deep gyrate erythema (non-pruritic, non-scaly, annular, red) (see **Figures 422–424**). Work-up includes a search for any antigenic stimulus, such as *Tinea pedis*, a new drug, blue-cheese ingestion (contains penicillin), streptococcal infection, thyroid disease, dental infection, viral infection (e.g. Epstein–Barr virus), or malignancy.

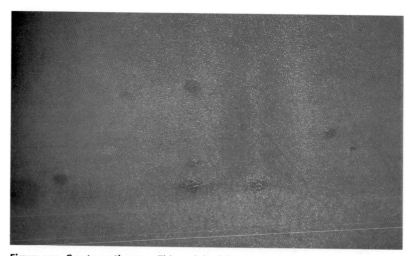

Figure 422. Gyrate erythema. This and the following two photographs were taken at approximately 3-week intervals and illustrate the deep variant of erythema annulare centrificum. The initial lesion is an erythematous, urticarial papule or plaque.

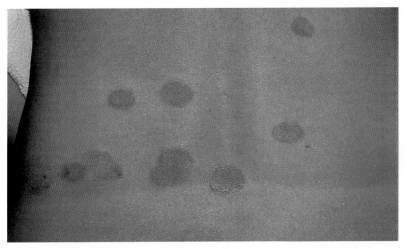

Figure 423. Gyrate erythema. By the third week, note how old lesions are bigger, some have coallesced, and new lesions have formed.

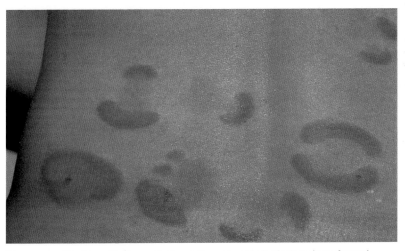

Figure 424. Gyrate erythema. By the sixth week, annular lesions have formed. Most lesions have had part of their circle resolved, leaving various arcs and post-inflammatory hyperpigmentation.

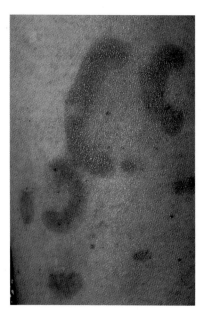

Figure 425. Jessner's lymphocytic infiltrate is a benign cutaneous dermatosis of unknown cause. Erythematous, red, non-scaly, infiltrated papules, plaques, and arcs on the face, arms, and trunk are characteristic. It is most common in adults, but may rarely affect children. Antinuclear antibody (ANA) and Ro (ss-A) autoantibody should be checked, and a biopsy performed.

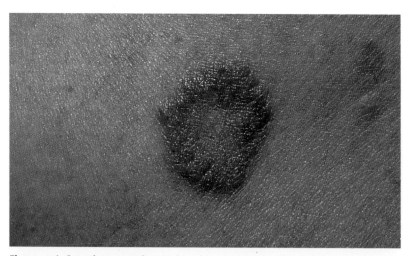

Figure 426. Granuloma annulare is thought to represent a delayed hypersensitivity reaction to as-yet unidentified cutaneous antigens. Initially, a red dermal papule forms and spreads outward, involuting centrally. Later, multiple dermal papules linked together form spreading, annular rings. Granuloma annulare is most common on the dorsa of the hands but lesions occur elsewhere (e.g. the elbows, fingers, palms, dorsa of the feet, etc.).

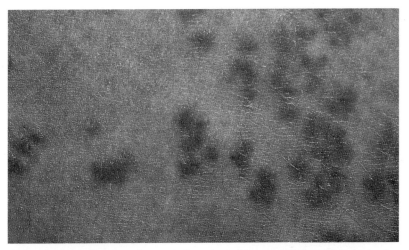

Figure 427. Granuloma annulare. A disseminated form, consisting of hundreds of papules and/or annular lesions spread across the trunk, may occur. It has been thought that the disseminated form of granuloma annulare is associated with diabetes, although a recent case-controlled study was not able to verify such an association.

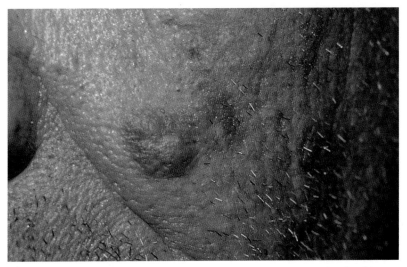

Figure 428. Granuloma faciale. Granuloma faciale is an uncommon localized form of a small-vessel vasculitis. It typically affects the face of middle-aged Caucasian people, particularly men. A red–brown plaque or plaques on the face, often with a peau d'orange surface, is characteristic. The nose is often involved.

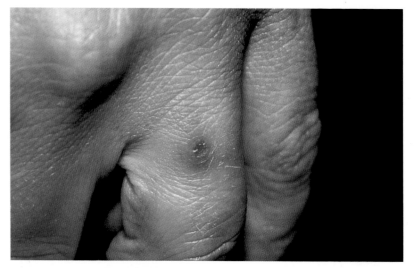

Figure 429. Foreign body, papule. Foreign bodies may produce inflammatory reactions in the skin. This patient presented with the solitary violaceous papule as shown. She denied a history of trauma.

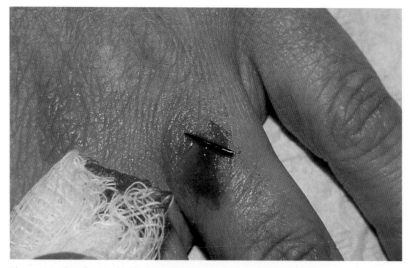

Figure 430. Foreign body, biopsy showing thorn. Only after biopsy and extraction of a thorn did the patient remember being 'stuck' by a Yucca plant 4–5 years before. To make the story even more surprising, the initial injury occurred 4–5 cm away on the dorsum of the hand.

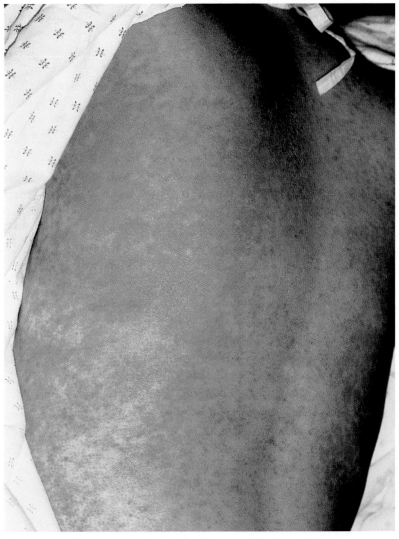

Figure 431. Graft versus host disease (GvHD) is a condition in which immunocompetent cells from transplanted tissue (usually an allogeneic bone marrow transplantation but less commonly a blood transfusion) attack the patient. It is typically divided into acute and chronic GvHD, with acute GvHD occurring within the first 3 months after transplantation, and chronic GvHD anytime thereafter. In acute GvHD, the patient typically presents between 7 and 21 days after grafting with a diffuse maculopapular erythematous eruption, although other patterns are possible, e.g. scarlatiniform or Stevens–Johnson like. Systemic symptoms include fever, hepatic dysfunction, and diarrhea. GvHD is often fatal. (Courtesy of Robert Sigafoes, MD)

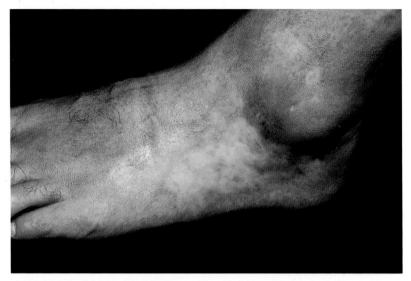

Figure 432. Graft versus host disease.   The skin lesions of chronic GvHD appear as lichenoid or sclerodermatous lesions (as shown). Over time, hypo- and hyperpigmentation, poikiloderma, sclerosis, alopecia, and ulceration may occur.

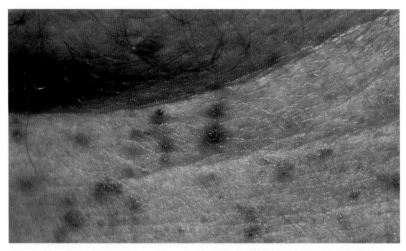

Figure 433. Grover's disease.   Grover's disease, also known as transient acantholytic dermatosis, is a type of 'heat rash' often associated with increased sweating. Women may develop it at menopause as a result of hot flashes. The patient should always be asked about increased sweating, particularly at night. One study showed it to be commonly associated with hospitalized patients on strict bed rest with abundant sweating. Discrete, truncal, pruritic papules and papulovesicles in a middle-aged or elderly person are characteristic. Although usually transient (weeks to months), the disease may also last years.

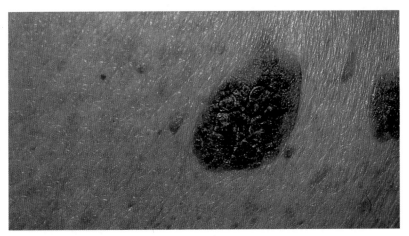

Figure 434. Seborrheic keratosis.   These brown, stuck-on, warty, papules or plaques are found on almost every older adult and have been called 'barnacles on the ship of life'. They may be dark brown or black, light tan or white, nearly flat or raised, smooth and greasy, or rough and warty. Almost any area of the body may be affected.

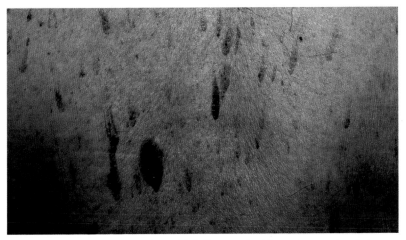

Figure 435. Seborrheic keratosis, multiple linear.   In older patients, seborrheic keratoses can be numerous, especially on the trunk. They may be linear in shape, as shown here.

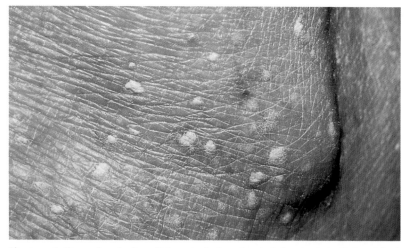

Figure 436. Stucco keratosis. This variant of a seborrheic keratosis is distinguished by its white color and preference for the tops of the feet and/or ankles in an older adult.

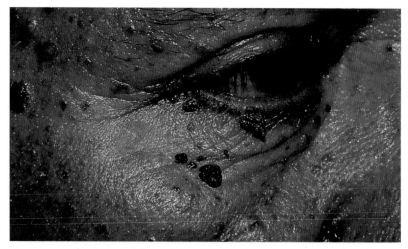

Figure 437. Dermatosis papulosa nigra is a common papular condition of the face and neck in darker-skinned patients. Multiple, pigmented papules, flat or filiform, are characteristic.

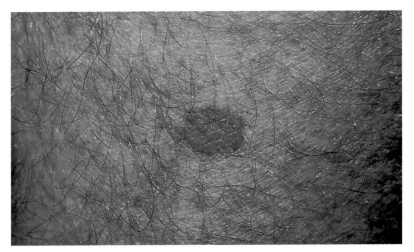

Figure 438. Benign lichenoid keratosis. The classic story is that of a brown spot, present for months to years, that suddenly becomes red, inflamed, slightly raised, and itchy. It is as if the body suddenly decides to go on the attack.

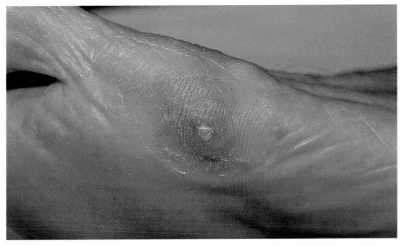

Figure 439. Corn. This hyperkeratotic, painful papule on the sole, dorsum of the toes, or in the web spaces is the result of repeated pressure. An underlying bony prominence or exostosis is always found. Direct pressure causes pain.

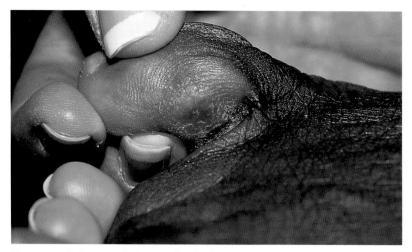

Figure 440. Soft corn. Soft corns develop in the interdigital spaces, usually between the 4th and 5th toes, and are so called because the hyperkeratotic skin is hydrated and soft.

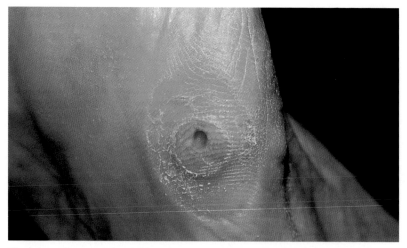

Figure 441. Corn, pared. Paring of a corn reveals the characteristic translucent core—in contrast to a wart, which shows black dots and bleeding (**Figure 442**).

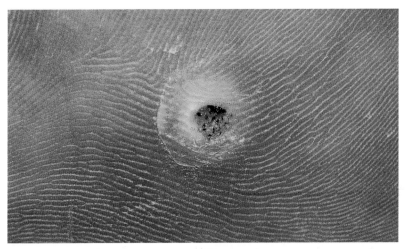

Figure 442. Verruca. In contrast to a corn (**Figure 441**), paring a verruca reveals black dots and bleeding. The black dots represent thrombosed capillaries. (See also **Figures 351–356**.)

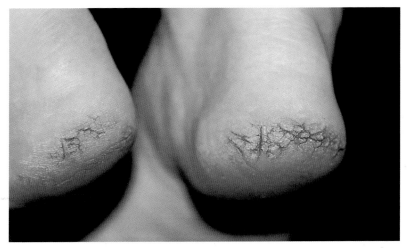

Figure 443. Hyperkeratosis of the heels. Hyperkeratosis beginning laterally, with potential progression to cover the entire heel, is common in middle-aged patients. Some have suggested that causes are faulty walking technique, pressure, sandals, and ill-fitting shoes.

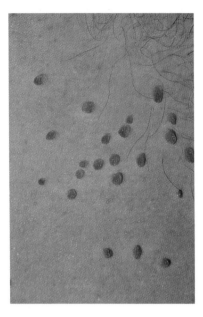

Figure 444. Skin tags. Pedunculated or filiform, fleshy, pink, or brown papules, 1–10 mm, on the sides of the neck, axilla, eyelids, or groin in a middle-aged or older adult are characteristic of skin tags, also called acrochordons. Patients often complain that tags on the neck catch on collars or necklaces. The presence of skin tags positively correlates with weight, height, and colonic polyps.

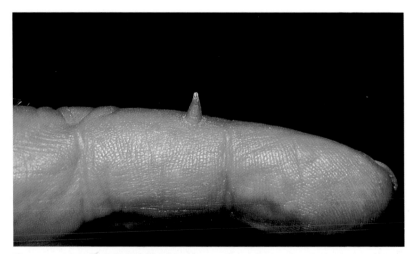

Figure 445. Acquired digital fibrokeratoma. These flesh-colored papules on the finger, usually index or middle finger, are characteristically mistaken for warts. One tell-tale feature that distinguishes it from a wart is an epidermal collarette at its base. These lesions may also occur on the toes, palms, or heels.

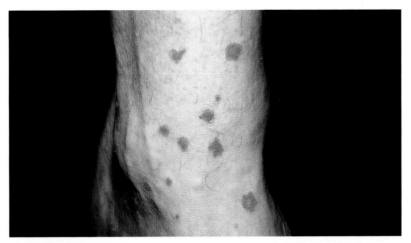

Figure 446. Disseminated superficial porokeratosis is a condition in which the patient develops multiple small, circular lesions each of which represents a spreading clone of abnormal cells. Clinically, one sees multiple, red or brown, oval or circular lesions on the extensor arms and legs of a middle-aged woman. A tiny continuous ridge runs along the edge of each lesion. Immunosuppression (e.g. HIV, transplantation) and ultraviolet light (e.g. sun bathing, PUVA, tanning booth) can either trigger or exacerbate this condition. Autosomal-dominant inheritance may occur, and the development of squamous cell carcinoma is an uncommon complication.

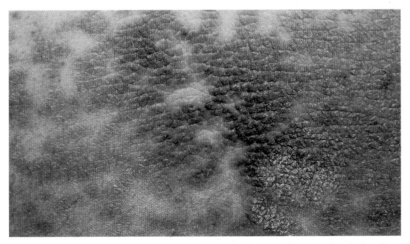

Figure 447. Confluent and reticulated papillomatosis. Confluent and reticulated papillomatosis presents in the mid-chest and axilla in young adults. Its cause is unknown. Confluent and reticulated brown papules may be found in the mid chest, back, neck, abdomen, axilla and inframammary area.

NAIL DISORDERS

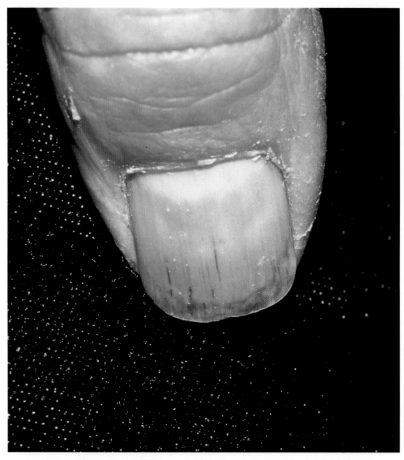

Figure 448. Splinter hemorrhage. A longitudinal, linear, red or black streak below the nail is characteristic. Common 'benign' splinter hemorrhages occur in the middle or distal nail bed and are black. They are common in elderly people. This contrasts with the rarer splinter hemorrhages associated with systemic disease (e.g. subacute bacterial endocarditis) that occur more proximally and are red.

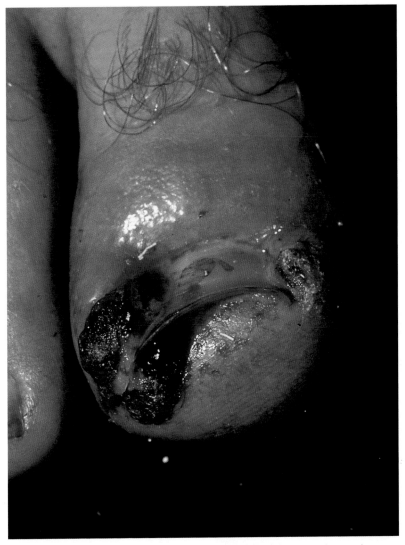

Figure 449. Ingrown nail. A swollen, red, lateral nailfold that extends over the lateral edge of the nail is characteristic. The nail burrows into the lesion, causing a foreign body response and producing more swelling. The big toe is most commonly affected. Secondary bacterial infection occurs.

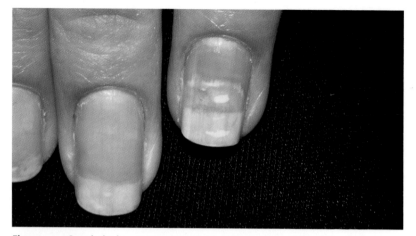

Figure 450. Onycholysis.   Separation of the nail plate from the bed is called onycholysis and is most commonly seen in women. Causes include psoriasis (look for pits, family history, oil spots), trauma (ask if they are cleaning under nails and with what?), photo-onycholysis (e.g. from tetracycline or less commonly psoralens), allergic contact dermatitis (from nail products such as hardeners or polish), systemic causes (e.g. thyroid abnormalities, pregnancy), and fungal infection (e.g. *Candida* species). Women with onycholysis of long fingernails and no other obvious cause may have developed them secondary to chronic lifting of the nail off the bed during the course of normal activity.

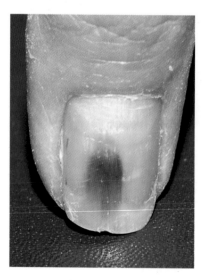

Figure 451. *Pseudomonas.* A green discoloration of the nail occurs when the space created by onycholysis is colonized by *Pseudomonas* species.

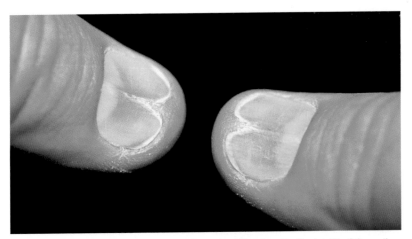

Figure 452. Median canalicular dystrophy.　A midline longitudinal split of the nail (usually the thumb nail) occurs in median canalicular dystrophy. Lines extending outward on both sides give the appearance of a fir tree.

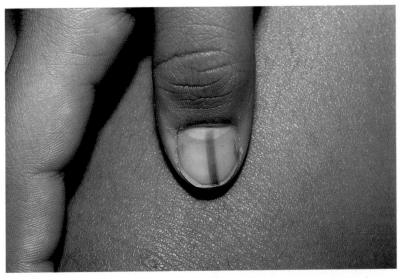

Figure 453. Longitudinal melanonychia, benign.　Any pigmentation of the nail matrix (just below the proximal nail fold) may give rise to a longitudinal pigmented band. A nevus is the usual cause, but an atypical nevus or a melanoma must be excluded. Benign lesions tend to be multiple, narrow bands uniformly colored, occurring in younger people, whereas malignant lesions tend to be solitary, wide, dark and/or multicolored in an older person. Pigmentation of the periungual skin (Hutchison's sign) is particularly ominous. The lesion shown here was a solitary, congenital, stable lesion in a 6-year-old. (See also **Figure 192**).

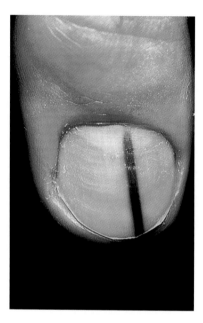

Figure 454. Longitudinal melanonychia, malignant. This solitary black streak developed in a young adult. Biopsy showed melanoma in situ.

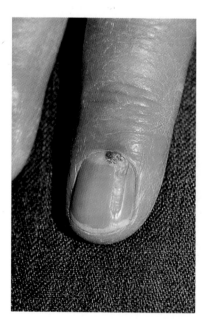

Figure 455. Digital mucous cyst, groove. A longitudinal groove of the nail plate may develop from any growth or tumor which pushes down on the nail matrix. The digital mucous cyst is most common, but a glomus tumor may be found as well.

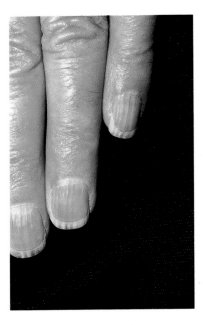

Figure 456. Nail ridges. Longitudinal ridges are so common in the older patient as to be considered normal.

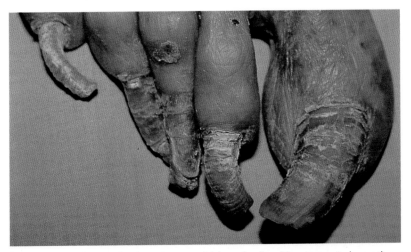

Figure 457. Onychogryphosis. Opaque, thickened nails with exaggerated growth upward and/or laterally are characteristic of nail hypertrophy. Old age and trauma are the primary causes. If the nails are permitted to grow, they may take on the appearance of a horn. This is called onychogryphosis. (Courtesy of Department of Dermatology, University of California, San Diego.)

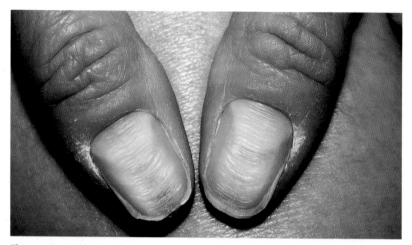

Figure 458. Habit tic deformity.   Chronic picking at the proximal nail fold can cause a dystrophy of the nail. Multiple transverse lines like a washboard are typical. Thickening of the skin at the proximal nail fold occurs as well, secondary to the chronic picking.

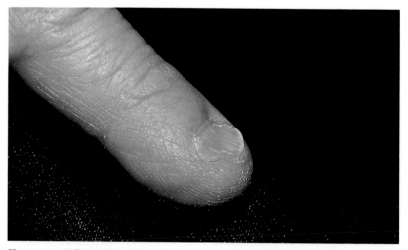

Figure 459. Koilonychia.   The nail is concave with the plate thinned and the edges everted in koilonychia, also known as spoon nails. It occurs not uncommonly in children on the hallux and may be familial. Associations include occupational trauma, Plummer–Vinson syndrome, iron deficiency anemia, and many others.

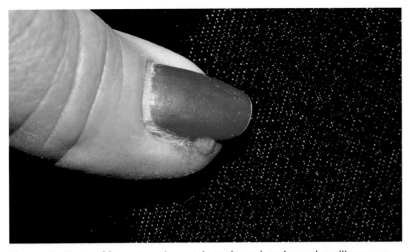

Figure 460. Paronychia, acute. An acutely tender, red, periungual swelling occurs in acute paronychia. Pus may be visible below the cuticle. The nail is usually not dystrophic. *Staphylococcus aureus* or *Streptococcus* species are the usual pathogens. Anaerobes and *Candida* species may also be found. Risk factors include trauma, manipulation, and isotretinoin.

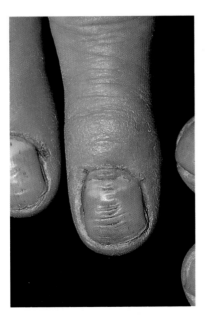

Figure 461. Paronychia, chronic. The periungual areas of multiple nails are swollen, red, and inflamed in chronic paronychia. The cuticle is lost and dystrophy of the nail often occurs. *Candida* species, *Proteus* species, *Klebsiella* species, *Staphylococcus* species, *Pseudomonas* species, and saprophytic fungi are potential pathogens. Risk factors include manicures, pushing back the cuticle, and frequent contact with water (e.g. housewives, bartenders). Several cases of immediate hypersensitivity to foods in food handlers have been reported to cause a chronic paronychia, as has allergic contact dermatitis to nail polish.

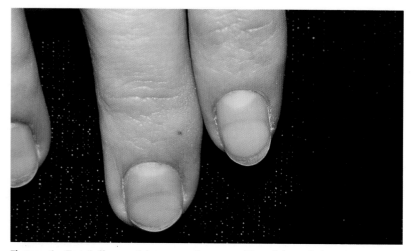

Figure 462. Beau's lines. A transverse furrow or ridge of the nail plate that develops after various diseases or chemotherapy is called a Beau's line. It is caused by temporary arrest of nail plate function. This patient had suffered from infectious mononucleosis 4 months before presentation.

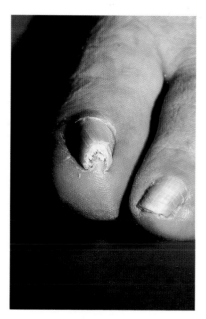

Figure 463. Pincer nail. A pincer nail is excessively curved. The nail bed is often 'drawn up' and pinched by the edges of the nail. Pain may be significant.

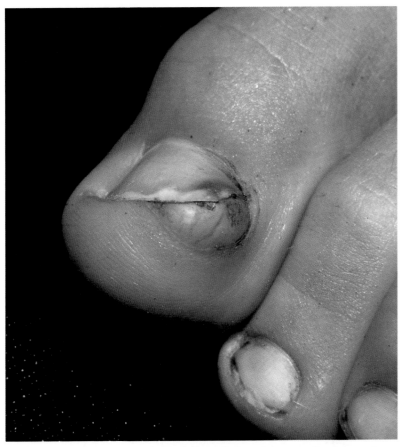

Figure 464. Exostosis. A firm subungual papule or nodule protruding from under the distal nail is characteristic. The dorsal, medial aspect of the hallux is the most common site. Dystrophy of the overlying nail plate may occur. Diagnosis is by X-ray. A benign osseous proliferation is the underlying cause.

See also onychomycosis (**Figure 323**), mucocutaneous candidiasis (**Figure 326**), proximal subungual onychomycosis (**Figure 282**), acral lentiginous melanoma (**Figure 496**), and Terry's nails (**Figure 595**).

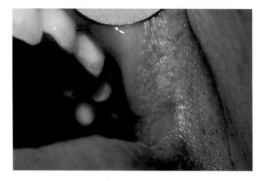

Figure 465. Fordyce spots.
These tiny, multiple, pinpoint, yellow papules on the lips or buccal mucosa represent ectopic sebaceous glands and are usually an incidental finding requiring no treatment.

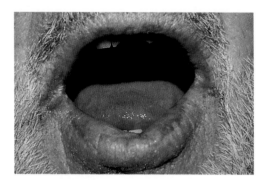

Figure 466. Perleche.
Redness, scaling, and crusting at the corner of the mouth occur in angular cheilitis, also known as perleche. This disease represents yet another type of intertrigo where body folds opposed keep the skin excessively moist and macerated. Bacteria and *Candida* species may cause secondary infection. Lip licking in the young, mouth breathing (day or night or related to orthodontic devices causing excessive saliva), and decreased vertical separation of the mandible and maxilla (e.g. in older patients from lack of teeth or bone resorption), causing a prominent skin fold, are all risk factors.

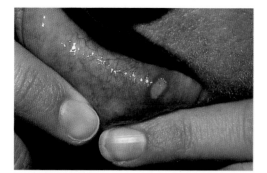

Figure 467. Aphthous ulcer. These shallow intraoral ulcers can be extremely painful and often come in crops. The grayish center is usually surrounded by a bright red halo. Extensive and painful aphthosis may occur in patients with HIV infection. Genital and oral ulceration associated with iritis occurs in Behçet's syndrome (see **Figures 367** and **368**).

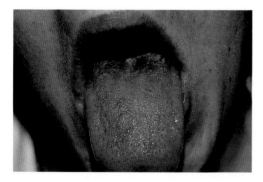

Figure 468. Black hairy tongue. The surface of the tongue is black, velvety, and hairlike in this unusual condition. Topical or oral antibiotics, poor oral hygiene, smoking, alcohol, or the use of mouthwashes may precipitate this condition.

See also pemphigus vulgaris (**Figure 204**), cicatricial pemphigoid (**Figure 212**), paraneoplastic pemphigus (**Figure 208**), geographic tongue (**Figure 543**), lichen planus (**Figures 550** and **551**).

PHOTODISTRIBUTED DISORDERS

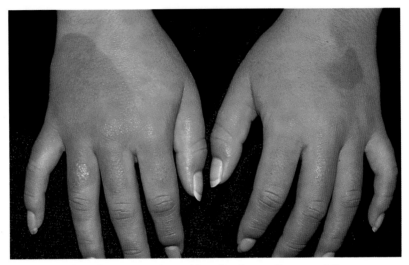

Figure 469. Phytophotocontact dermatitis. Burning, erythema, and, if severe, bulla formation followed by dark post-inflammatory hyperpigmentation distributed in bizarre linear arrangements are characteristic. The cause is furocoumarins in plants or fruit, which when inadvertently placed in contact with the skin, make it photosensitive. Common offenders include oranges, limes, lemons, celery, figs, dill, carrots, and parsley. This patient squeezed limes in preparing tropical drinks at an outdoor party. (See **Figure 512**.)

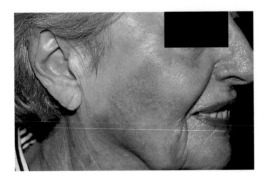

Figure 470. Photoallergic contact dermatitis. This woman's facial erythema resulted from a photocontact reaction with an ingredient in her moisturizer. Sunscreens are currently one of the most common causes of photoallergy. It is believed that ultraviolet light alters the compound, creating an allergen to which the patient reacts.

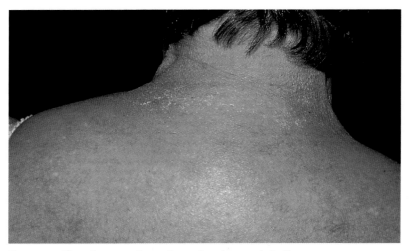

Figure 471. Photodrug eruption. Drugs that characteristically cause photosensitivity include NSAIDs, quinacrine (as shown here), doxycycline, and thiazides.

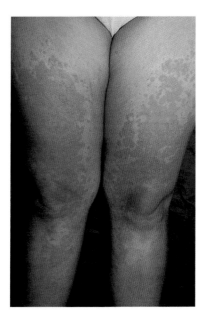

Figure 472. Polymorphous light eruption. Several hours after sun exposure, patients may develop papulovesicular, urticarial, papular or plaque-type lesions. The face and neck are not typically affected, as these areas, through regular exposure, harden to the sun's effects. Outbreaks occur in the summer and may affect any photoexposed area. Patients who travel to sun-intense areas for brief vacations may be most severely affected. Antinuclear antibody (ANA) and Ro (SS-A) should be obtained to exclude lupus erythematosus.

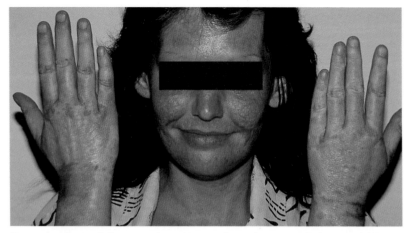

Figure 473. Systemic lupus erythematosus. Several patterns of photosensitivity may occur in lupus erythematosus. Bilateral erythema of the cheeks and malar eminences (butterfly rash) and/or a more extensive photodistributed rash may be seen in systemic lupus erythematosus (SLE) (see also **Figure 217**). Discoid lesions that are more fixed and discrete tend to occur in photoexposed areas such as the face, scalp, and upper trunk in both disseminated lupus erythematosus (see **Figures 219** and **220**) and SLE. Finally, photodistributed papulosquamous or annular lesions may occur in subacute cutaneous lupus erythematosus (**Figures 222** and **223**).

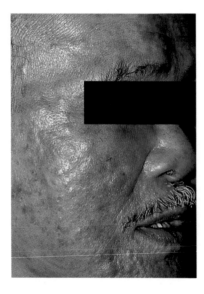

Figure 474. Chronic actinic dermatosis is a photosensitivity dermatitis that gives rise to erythematous and eczematous lesions. Elderly men, patients with HIV infection, and recently some patients with atopic dermatitis have been identified. The term chronic actinic dermatitis has been proposed as the unifying term for photosensitivity dermatitis, actinic reticuloid, persistent light reactivity, and photosensitive eczema. Persistent erythema of the face in a middle-aged to elderly person is characteristic. With time, the skin may become eczematous and lichenified, and a leonine facies may result. Although histologic features may suggest a lymphoma, chronic actinic dermatosis is not a premalignant condition. For unclear reasons, these patients have a high incidence of contact allergy sensitivity to plant oleoresin extracts, fragrances, and lichens.

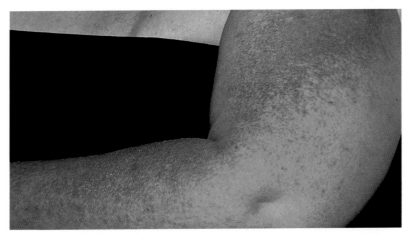

Figure 475. Dermatomyositis.   The erythematous rash of dermatomyositis often occurs in a photosensitive distribution, commonly affecting the upper back and chest as well as the photoexposed areas of the arms. Other characteristic changes include periorbital edema and red, scaly papules over the knuckles. (See also **Figures 224** and **225**.)

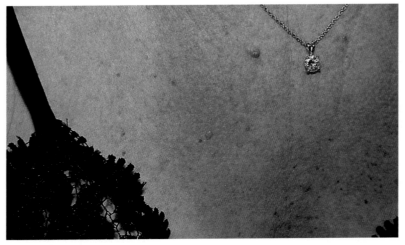

Figure 476. Solar urticaria.   Urticarial plaques developing within minutes and in the exact distribution of sun exposure are characteristic of solar urticaria. Systemic symptoms including syncope may occur. The lesions usually resolve within hours. ANA, Ro and La should be negative.

NEVI AND MELANOMA

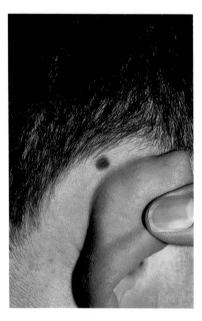

Figure 477. Benign nevus, junctional. Common, acquired nevi begin appearing in the first year of life. They grow in size and number, peaking in the third or fourth decade. They are most common above the waist on the sun-exposed skin. Initially, nevi tend to be flat and dark as shown here in a child. Over time, they become raised. At some point during adulthood, many nevi lose their color and appear as flesh-colored papules (**Figure 478**).

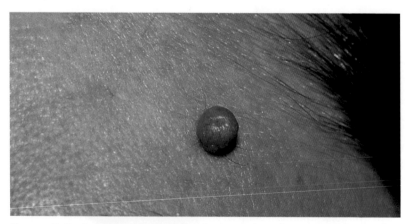

Figure 478. Benign nevus, intradermal. Benign nevi may be categorized generally as flat and pigmented (junctional) (**Figure 477**), raised and pigmented (compound), or raised and flesh-colored (dermal) as shown here.

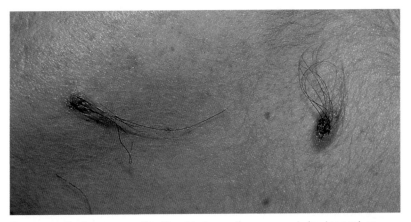

Figure 479. Benign nevus. Significant hair growth may occur in benign nevi, as illustrated here.

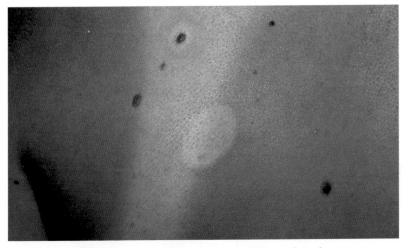

Figure 480. Halo nevus. The immune system in a child may, for unknown reasons, pick a mole to 'attack'. In the process, a surrounding ring of pigment is lost. Vitiligo may occasionally be found in the same patient. A halo nevus, like any other, should be evaluated by the ABCD criteria (see **Figure 489**) and, if atypical, removed. If left alone, the mole will shrink up and disappear over several years. A halo nevus is seen in the upper middle of the photograph. In the center, a halo is left as its mole has been 'removed' by the immune system. Note also that the right half of this halo is erythematous, being sunburned instead of tanned because of its lack of pigment.

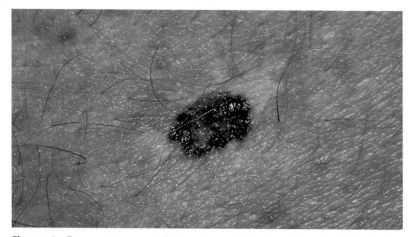

Figure 481. Recurrent nevus.   A benign pigmented lesion with atypical clinical and histologic features may develop in the scar of a partially removed nevus. Melanoma, however, must always be considered.

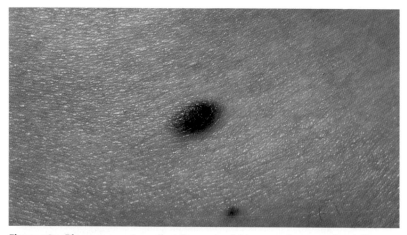

Figure 482. Blue nevus.   A small, solitary, round, blue macule or papule on the dorsum of the hands is characteristic of a blue nevus. It may also occur on the scalp or feet. A nodular type occasionally occurs on the buttocks. The brown pigment of the dermis looks blue because of the Tyndall effect. The Tyndall effect is the preferential absorption of long wavelengths of light by melanin and the scattering of shorter wavelengths, representing the blue end of the spectrum, by collagen bundles.

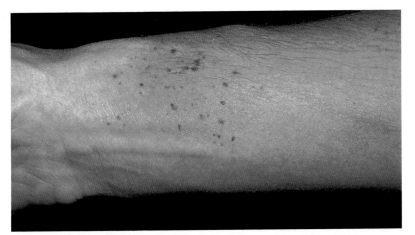

Figure 483. Nevus spilus. A tan patch speckled with brown or black spots is typical. Onset is usually in childhood or adolescence. Lesions are typically 1–5 cm in size but rarely may be much larger. In some lesions, the background tan color is absent. Very rarely, malignant change may occur.

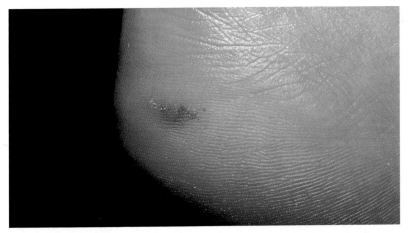

Figure 484. Talon noire, or black heel, is characterized by tiny black pinpoint dots grouped together and located somewhere along the posterior edge of the heel. The patients are usually athletically involved in sports such as basketball, soccer, volleyball, etc. Sheer forces causing extravasation of blood are thought to be the cause. The lesion is most commonly confused with a verruca and occasionally a melanoma. A similar change may occur on the palmar aspect of the fingers.

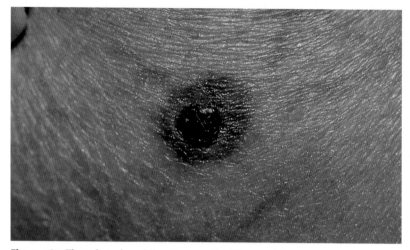

Figure 485. Thrombosed angiokeratoma. A solitary angiokeratoma may thrombose, with the resultant lesion resembling a melanoma.

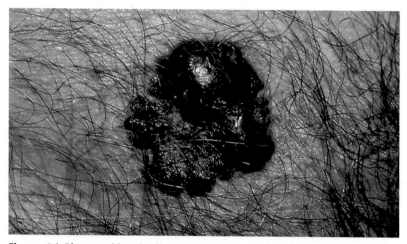

Figure 486. Pigmented basal cell carcinoma. Occasionally, a basal cell carcinoma may retain enough pigment to mimic a melanoma. (See also **Figure 631**.) (Courtesy of Department of Dermatology, University of California, San Diego.)

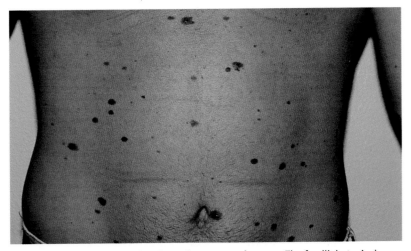

Figure 487. Familial atypical mole–melanoma syndrome. The familial atypical mole–melanoma syndrome (FAM–M syndrome) combines a personal or family history of melanoma with multiple clinically atypical nevi. These patients often have a large number of nevi (e.g. >50) as well as nevi in unusual sites, e.g. the buttocks, dorsa of the feet, anterior aspect of the scalp, etc. Patients should be monitored closely, as their risk for developing melanoma is high.

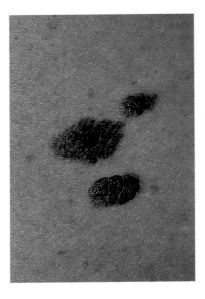

Figure 488. Familial atypical mole–melanoma syndrome. Close-up examination shows nevi with irregular borders, diameter >6 mm, and irregular colors.

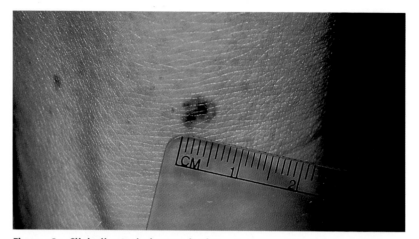

Figure 489. Clinically atypical nevus, benign. Every new dermatologic patient should be encouraged to have a complete skin examination. Return patients should have one every 2–3 years. Monthly self-examination should also be encouraged. All pigmented lesions should be evaluated by the ABCD criteria as follows. Any lesion with two of the following should be termed a clinically atypical nevus and removed for histologic examination: (i) **a**symmetric shape, (ii) irregular **b**order, (iii) variegated **c**olor, and (iv) **d**iameter greater than 6 mm. Although irregular in shape and containing multiple colors, this lesion was benign.

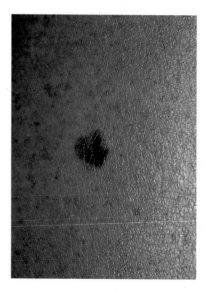

Figure 490. Clinically atypical nevus— melanoma in situ. If the lesion fulfils the histologic criteria for melanoma but is confined to the epidermis, the term melanoma in situ is used. At this initial stage, there is no possibility of metastatic spread.

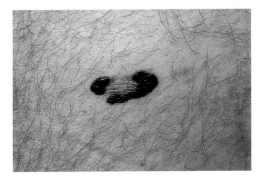

Figure 491. Melanoma in situ with regression.
The immune system fights a war with the neoplasm, trying to destroy it. It may be successful in portions of the lesion, and this is called regression. Regression appears as a lack of pigment, as shown here in the center of the lesion.

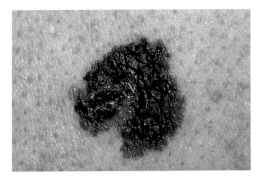

Figure 492. Melanoma, superficial spreading.
All the ABCD criteria are fulfilled here. The lesion is large, irregular in shape, border, and color. Risk factors for melanoma include the presence of one or more of the following: clinically atypical (formerly called dysplastic) nevi, increased number of nevi, family history of melanoma, increased propensity to sunburn, a tendency to freckle, and blond or red hair.

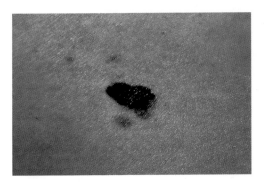

Figure 493. Melanoma.
Melanomas may arise from normal skin or from a pre-existing nevus as shown here.

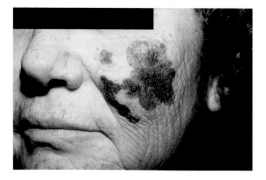

Figure 494. Lentigo maligna melanoma. A slowly enlarging, irregularly pigmented, irregularly shaped macule on the sun-exposed skin of an older adult is characteristic. A Wood's light may be helpful in delineating the extent of the lesion. Histologically, lentigo maligna remains confined to the epidermis. When invasion into the dermis occurs, the term lentigo maligna melanoma is used. (Courtesy of Michael O Murphy, MD)

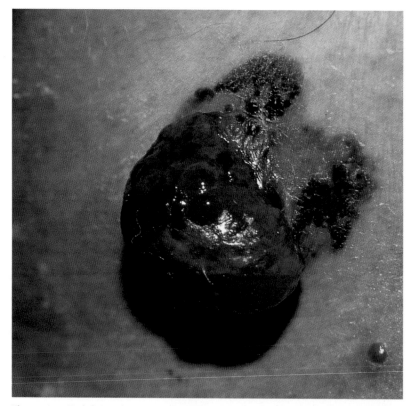

Figure 495. Nodular melanoma. A melanoma may occasionally present as a rapidly growing nodule. It may be brown or black or relatively devoid of pigment, as shown here. Any focus of pigment within a vascular lesion should arouse suspicion.

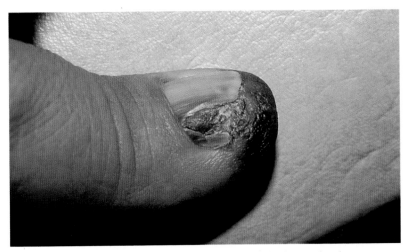

Figure 496. Acral lentiginous melanoma. The so-called subungual melanoma probably begins in the nail matrix and presents initially as longitudinal melanonychia (see **Figures 453** and **454**). As the melanoma spreads, nail destruction may occur, with pigment extending to the proximal nail fold (Hutchison's sign) or to the fingertip.

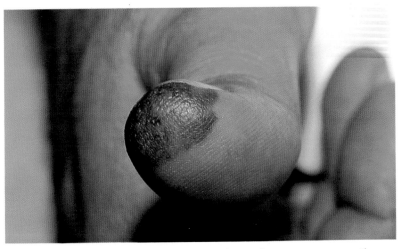

Figure 497. Acral lentiginous melanoma. Rarely, a melanoma may occur on the palms, soles, fingers, or toes. When dark-skinned patients develop melanoma, this is the most common type.

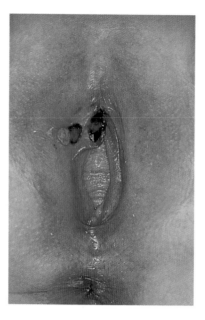

Figure 498. Melanoma, vulva.
Benign nevi, vulvar melanosis, and melanoma may occur in the vulvar region. Any pigmented lesion should be evaluated for irregularity in shape or color and biopsied if indicated. The patient shown developed her melanoma at 75 years of age. (Courtesy of Paul Koonings, MD.)

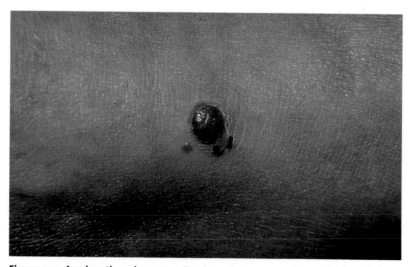

Figure 499. Amelanotic melanoma.   Rarely, melanomas may be totally devoid of pigment, making the diagnosis very difficult. This vascular papule on the ankle of a 22-year-old woman was thought to be a hemangioma.

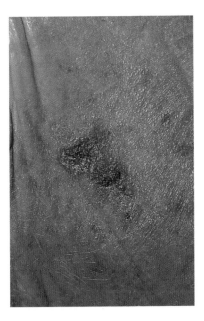

Figure 500. Amelanotic lentigo maligna. In very rare cases, a lentigo maligna may be devoid of pigment. The correct diagnosis is rarely suspected. This red scaly lesion was thought to represent Bowen's disease or a basal cell carcinoma. Only after two biopsies was the correct diagnosis believed.

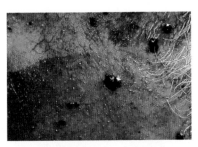

Figure 501. Metastatic melanoma, pigmented. Melanomas may recur at the surgical site, in transit to regional lymph nodes or at distant sites. Multiple pigmented cutaneous lesions may occur as shown. Diffuse hyperpigmentation and melanuria can develop rarely. (Photograph courtesy of Department of Dermatology, University of California, San Diego.)

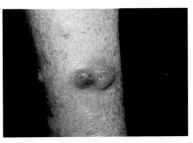

Figure 502. Metastatic melanoma, red. Any new cutaneous growth in a patient with a history of melanoma should be considered as a possible metastatic focus. This patient developed multiple nodules of metastatic melanoma on the leg near the site of the initial melanoma.

See also spitz nevus (**Figure 106**).

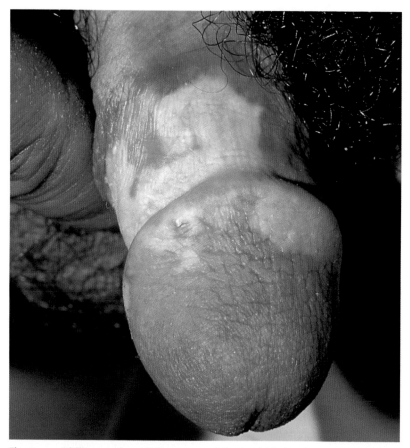

Figure 503. Vitiligo, penis.   Vitiligo is a condition in which the skin loses its color in well-defined patches. It occurs in about 1–2% of the world's population. A family history is present in about 20–30% of cases and is more commonly seen in patients with younger onset of the disease. It seems to represent an autoimmune condition in which the patient's immune system attacks the pigment-producing cells (i.e. melanocytes). Peak onset is 10–30 years of age. Patients with onset over 40 years of age should have a complete skin examination to exclude coexistent melanoma. Various autoimmune diseases are associated, with demonstration of autoantibodies typical (e.g. thyroid). Sharply depigmented, often symmetric patches occurring anywhere, but with preference for the face, fingers, trunk, and extremities, result. A chemical leukoderma from industrial exposure to hydroquinones, catechols, phenols, or mercaptoamines is rare but occurs and can be indistinguishable from vitiligo.

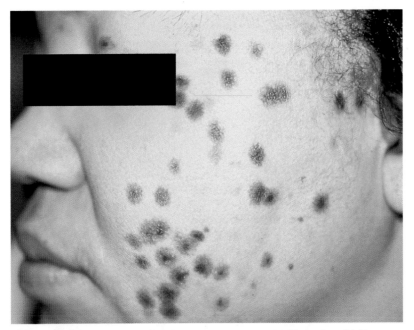

Figure 504. Vitiligo, diffuse. This African-American patient has severe vitiglio; the dark spots are actually the patient's normal skin color. Such diffuse loss of pigmentation can be psychologically devastating. (Courtesy of Theodore Sebastien, MD.)

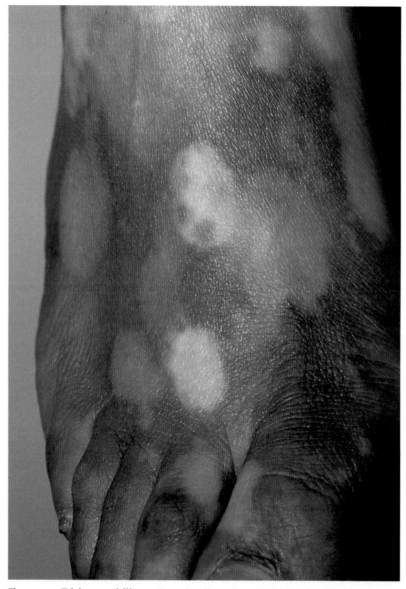

Figure 505. Trichrome vitiligo. Occasionally, an intermediate color may be present, making the patient 'three-colored'.

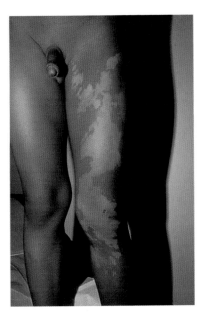

Figure 506. Segmental vitiligo. In this distinct variant of vitiligo, an acquired depigmented patch of skin in a segmental or dermatomal pattern occurs. In contrast to the typical vitiligo, new lesions cease after 1 year, onset is in childhood in the majority, Köbnerization does not occur, halo nevi are not associated, and response to psoralen plus ultraviolet light photochemotherapy is poor. (Courtesy of Michael O Murphy, MD.)

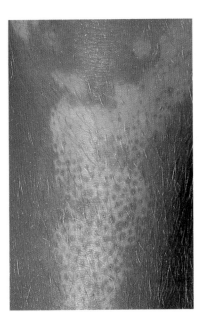

Figure 507. Follicular repigmentation of vitiligo. When vitiligo repigments, it often does so initially about the hair follicles.

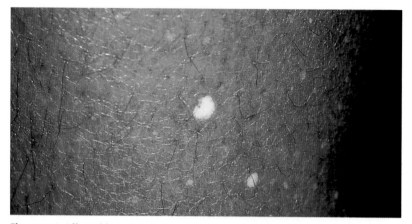

Figure 508. Idiopathic guttate hypomelanosis. Multiple, white macules, usually 1–4 mm in diameter, symmetrically distributed on the outer forearms or extensor legs are characteristic. Women are more commonly affected than men, as are people over 40 years of age. The cause is unknown.

See also post-inflammatory hypopigmentation (**Figure 129**), steroid hypo-pigmentation (**Figure 202**) and halo nevi (**Figure 480**).

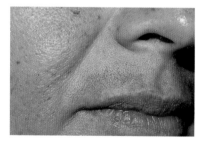

Figure 509. Melasma is a benign hyperpigmentation of the sun exposed skin of the face, typically seen in a woman. The combination of female hormones (e.g. pregnancy, oral contraceptives) and the sun combine to cause this disease. Symmetric, uniformly hyperpigmented, sharply defined macules and patches on the face in the sun-exposed areas result. It commonly affects the upper lip, cheeks, and forehead. Although both sexes and all races may be affected, women with darker skin predominate.

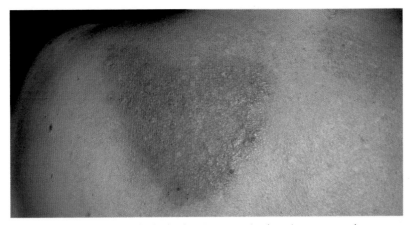

Figure 510. Macular amyloidosis, back. Degenerating keratinocytes may be converted in the dermis to a pigmented substance called amyloid. When this occurs, the skin takes on a brownish color. A habit of scratching is often found and may be carried out with a variety of instruments including the fingers, back scratchers, towels, or a nylon brush. The dark brown patches may have a reticulated or rippled pattern. Middle-aged, dark-skinned patients are commonly affected.

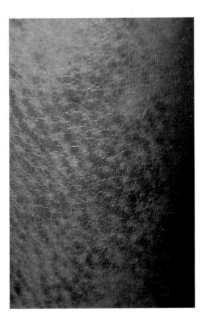

Figure 511. Lichen amyloidosis, shins. When the lesions of amyloid are palpable, the term lichen amyloidosis is used. Scratching or some type of rubbing is always present, which is presumed to be the cause of the thickening of the skin. Non-palpable macular amyloid may also occur. Many patients have other diseases associated with pruritus, e.g. atopy, stasis dermatitis. Note the uniformity of the color and the rippled pattern.

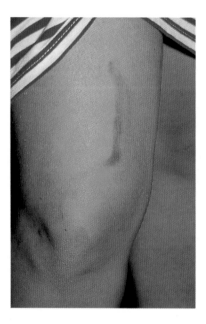

Figure 512. Phytophotocontact dermatitis. Burning, erythema, and, when severe, bulla formation, followed by dark post-inflammatory hyperpigmentation distributed in bizarre linear arrangements are characteristic. (See also **Figure 469**.)

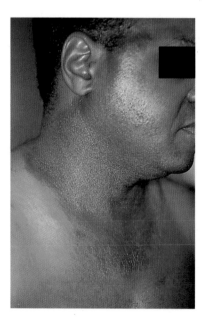

Figure 513. Post-inflammatory hyperpigmentation. Dark patches may develop after almost any disturbance of the skin in a dark-skinned patient. This patient had experienced an allergic contact dermatitis to a cologne. (Courtesy of Steven Goldberg, MD.)

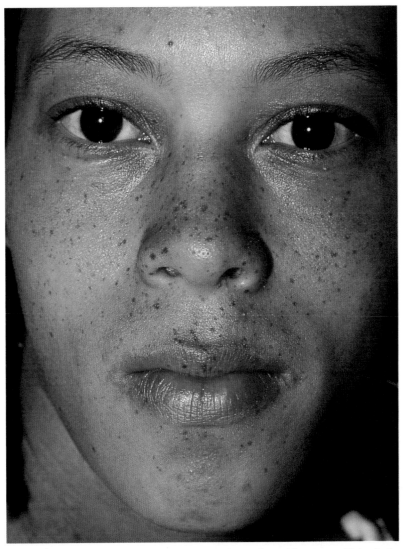

Figure 514. Patterned inherited lentiginosis.   This patient with patterned inherited lentiginosis has a striking lentiginous pigmentation of the central face and lips without mucous membrane or internal involvement. Lentigines may also be seen elsewhere, e.g. the buttocks or elbows. Inheritance is autosomal dominant. No systemic abnormalities are associated. Darker-skinned patients are most commonly affected.

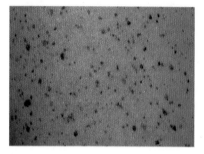

Figure 515. Leopard syndrome.
This mnemonic stands for **l**entigines, **e**lectrocardiogram abnormalities, **o**cular hypertelorism, **p**ulmonary stenosis, **a**bnormal genitalia, **r**etardation of growth, and **d**eafness. The darkly pigmented freckles or lentigines begin in infancy and progress. There is an autosomal dominant inheritance pattern. Only some of the non-cutaneous findings may be present in any one patient. An electrocardiogram should always be obtained.

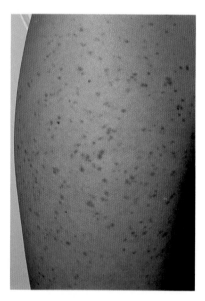

Figure 516. Urticaria pigmentosa.
Various patterns of cutaneous mastocytosis occur. In urticaria pigmentosa, multiple, brown macules or papules occur scattered on the body. Patients may have a few to several thousand. The pigmentation histologically is basal melanosis. See also **Figures 103–105**.

See also Peutz–Jeghers syndrome, **Figure 57**.

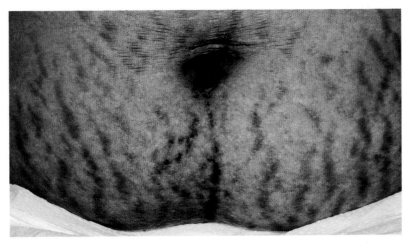

Figure 517. Linea nigra. Various pigmentary changes may occur in pregnancy, including the development of linea nigra (shown here), melasma (**Figure 509**), and pigmentary demarcation lines, as well as a generalized darkening of the skin which is particularly prominent in the areola and genitalia. Linea nigra is defined as a linear streak running vertically along the midline of the abdomen from the symphysis pubis to the xyphoid process. Striae distensae, which commonly develop in pregnancy, are also shown. The pigmentary changes of pregnancy usually fade over 6–12 months.

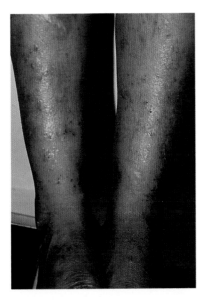

Figure 518. Pruritus in pregnancy. A significant percentage of pregnant women may develop pruritus during pregnancy. One must always rule out non-pregnancy-related causes such as scabies, xerosis, atopic dermatitis, etc. Potential pregnancy-related causes include cholestasis and early pemphigoid gestationis. The majority, however, fall into a broad and poorly defined category, as did this patient. Most of her skin changes are from scratching.

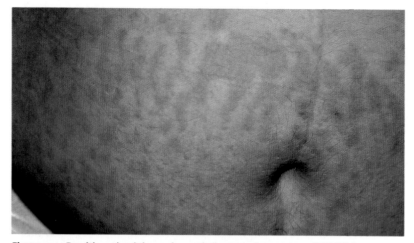

Figure 519. Pruritic urticarial papules and plaques of pregnancy (PUPPP) is a common itchy rash of pregnancy. It occurs principally in primigravidas in the third trimester. Urticarial, papular, and polycyclic lesions classically begin in the abdominal striae (as shown here) and abdomen but then may spread to the trunk, arms, thighs, and buttocks. PUPPP does not routinely flare postpartum as does herpes gestationis and has no tendency to recur in subsequent pregnancies. Direct immunofluorescence is negative. (Courtesy of Steven Goldberg, MD.)

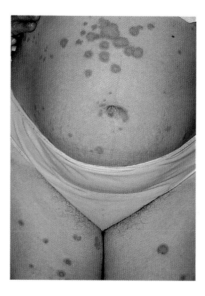

Figure 520. Pemphigoid gestationis, urticarial plaques. Pemphigoid gestationis (also known as herpes gestationis) is an autoimmune blistering disorder most commonly associated with pregnancy, although it may occur in association with trophoblastic tumors, hydatidiform mole, or choriocarcinoma. The skin lesions of pemphigoid gestationis often begin on the abdomen and include urticarial plaques and vesicles. Onset is usually in the second and third trimester but may occur in the first trimester or immediately postpartum. The neonate has skin lesions in approximately 5–10% of cases. Despite the name herpes gestationis, this rare pruritic subepidermal bullous eruption of pregnancy is unrelated to any viral infection.

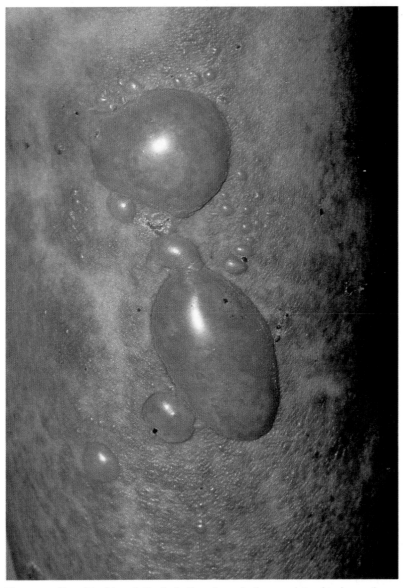

Figure 521. Pemphigoid gestationis, bulla. Large bullae may later develop, as in this patient who was experiencing a postpartum flare.

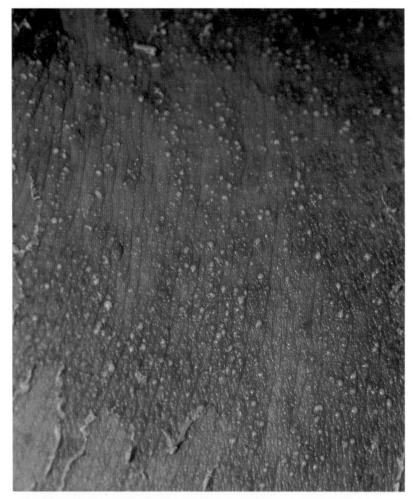

Figure 522. Impetigo herpetiformis. This disease has been called pustular psoriasis of pregnancy because of its clinical and histological resemblance to psoriasis, although no personal or family history of psoriasis is usually found. Superficial pustules studded on the periphery of erythematous plaques are characteristic. Hypocalcemia may be a precipitating factor, with tetany and convulsions. Stillbirths, placental insufficiency, and perinatal death are associated fetal complications.

See also spider angioma (**Figure 90**) and telogen effluvium (**Figure 268**).

PSORIASIS, LICHEN PLANUS, AND RELATED DISORDERS

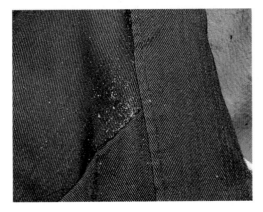

Figure 523. Dandruff.
The term dandruff applies to excessive scaling of the scalp. Pruritus is common. Inflammation and erythema are absent. Anyone will develop this condition if they shampoo infrequently enough.

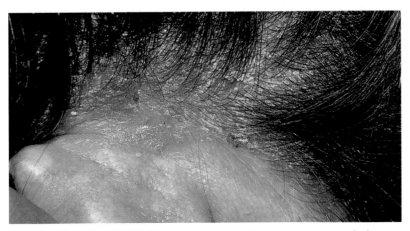

Figure 524. Seborrheic dermatitis. The term seborrheic dermatitis is used when some degree of inflammation and erythema is associated with scale in the seborrheic areas: the scalp, face, and trunk. The hair itself is unaffected. Overgrowth of the lipophilic yeast *Pityrosporum ovale* has been hypothesized as the etiologic agent.

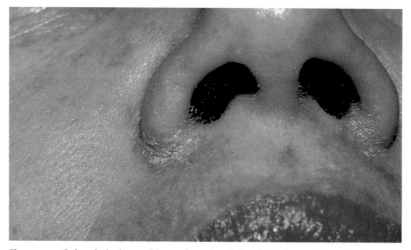

Figure 525. Seborrheic dermatitis, perinasal. Seborrheic dermatitis not only affects the scalp, but also the eyebrows, nasolabial folds, and midchest. Significant redness and scale of the nasolabial folds are seen here.

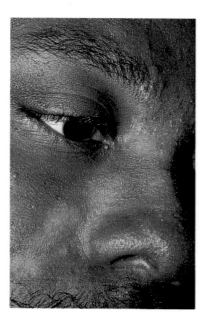

Figure 526. Seborrheic dermatitis is more common in dark-skinned patients because they tend to shampoo infrequently. Significant post-inflammatory hypopigmentation may occur.

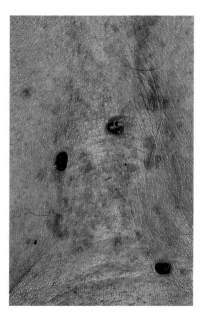

Figure 527. Seborrheic dermatitis, chest.
The red, scaly midchest in this adult man is typical of seborrheic dermatitis.

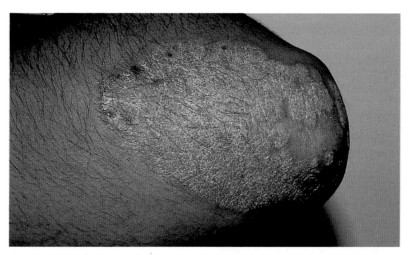

Figure 528. Psoriasis, papulosquamous plaque.   Psoriasis affects 1–2% of the population. The classic lesion is a sharply demarcated, raised, red plaque, covered with silvery-white scale. The elbows, knees, scalp, and intergluteal cleft are frequently involved. Köbnerization is typical. The disease tends to be chronic with periodic flares.

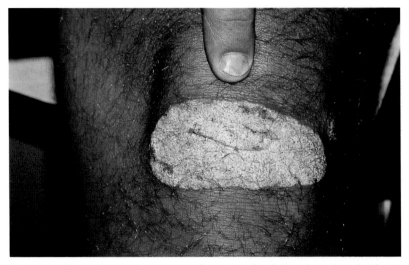

Figure 529. Psoriasis, papulosquamous plaque. A familial tendency is typical but other factors are also involved. Various drugs (e.g. beta-blockers), stress, or a streptococcal infection may precipitate a flare.

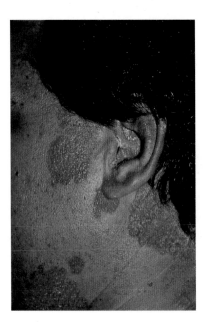

Figure 530. Psoriasis, scalp.
Scalp psoriasis — like seborrheic dermatitis — manifests itself as redness and scaling of the scalp. However, the crust is thicker, the lesions are better-defined and they are often more resistant to treatment. A plaque of redness and scale encircling the scalp, extending 1–2 cm beyond the hairline, is also characteristic and is shown here.

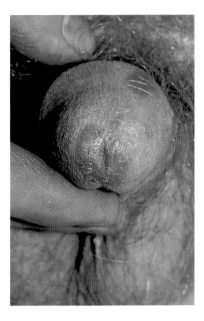

Figure 531. Psoriasis, penis.
The genitalia of both men and women are commonly involved.

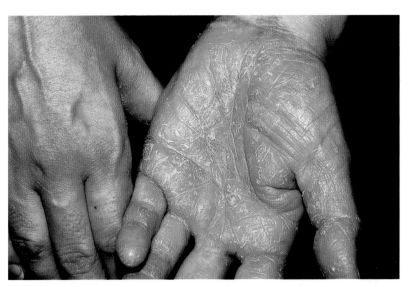

Figure 532. Psoriasis, palms. Plaque-type psoriasis of the palms may be particularly disabling. It may start out patchy, but often involves the entire palmar surface with redness, inflammation, and scale. Other forms of psoriasis that affect the palms and fingers are palmoplantar pustulosis (**Figure 540**) and acrodermatitis continua of Hallopeau (**Figure 541**).

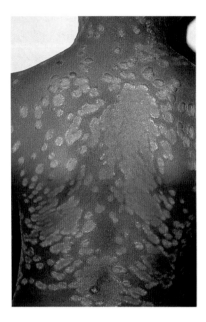

Figure 533. Psoriasis, dark-skinned child.   Psoriasis in a dark-skinned patient often leads to significant post-inflammatory hypopigmentation, as shown here.

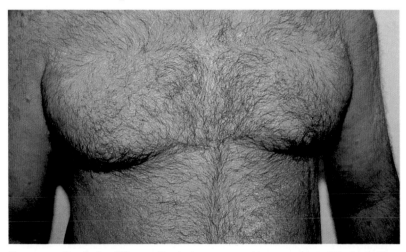

Figure 534. Psoriasis, diffuse.   Psoriasis may spread to cover most of the body. The extent of involvement is usually measured by calculating the percentage of total body surface area affected.

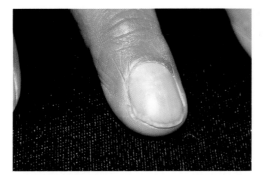

Figure 535. Psoriasis, nail pitting. Approximately half of patients with psoriasis may show nail involvement. When the matrix is involved, pits may form as shown here.

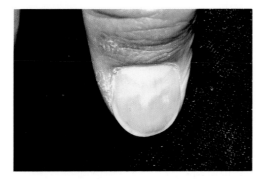

Figure 536. Psoriasis, oil spot. A yellow–brown subungual discoloration in a patient with psoriasis indicates involvement of the nail bed.

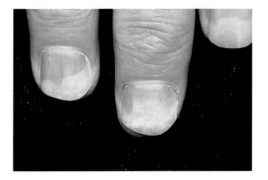

Figure 537. Psoriasis, onycholysis. If the nail bed is affected, onycholysis (separation of the nail plate from the bed) may occur.

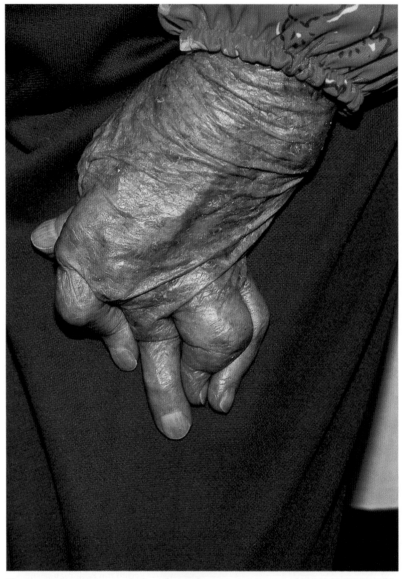

Figure 538. Psoriasis, psoriatic arthropathy. Various forms of seronegative arthritis occur in patients with psoriasis. The joints of the hands and fingers are most frequently involved, often with nail damage. Severe bone and joint destruction may occur, as shown here.

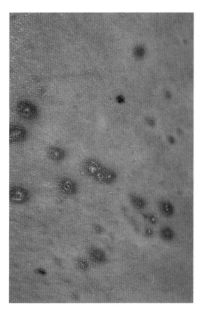

Figure 539. Psoriasis, guttate type.
The sudden development of disseminated 0.5–2.0 cm, red, scaly papules or small plaques is characteristic of acute, guttate (drop-shaped) psoriasis. A streptococcal infection is a very common precipitant. Children with psoriasis most often have this form. Spontaneous remission may occur or the disease may evolve into chronic plaque-type psoriasis. (See also **Figures 128** and **129**.)

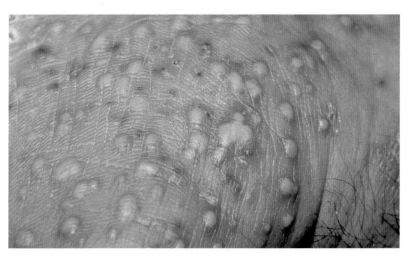

Figure 540. Palmoplantar pustulosis.   The periodic development of multiple pustules on the palms and/or soles is characteristic. Often the pustules do not rupture but instead turn brown. The course is chronic. An arthrosteitis has been associated and may be manifested by painful episodes of the anterior chest wall and, less commonly, the knee, spine, and ankle. Smoking is strongly associated.

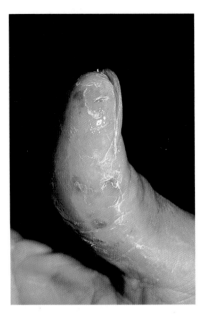

Figure 541. Acrodermatitis continua of Hallopeau is a variant of pustular psoriasis with a peculiar localization to the distal fingers. Sterile pustules on one or more fingers and fingertips that rupture, leaving tender, eroded skin, are characteristic. In the chronic stages, the skin may take on a papulosquamous appearance.

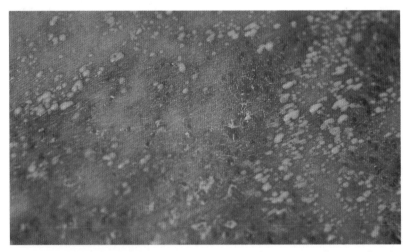

Figure 542. Psoriasis, pustular. In generalized pustular psoriasis of von Zumbusch, fever, generalized erythema, and pustules develop acutely. Erythematous plaques with pustules at the periphery are also characteristic. Hypoalbuminemia, hypocalcemia, loss of intravascular fluid, and renal failure are potential complications.

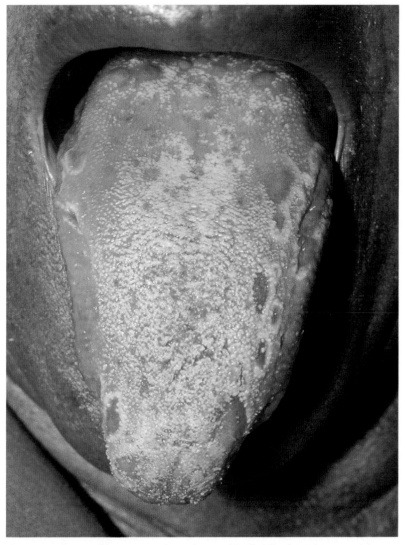

Figure 543. Geographic tongue.   Smooth, atrophic, 'bald' red patches or annular, serpiginous, white, yellow lines occur in geographic tongue, also known as benign migratory glossitis or glossitis areata migrans. Combinations of the two forms occur. This condition is 4–5 times more prevalent in psoriatic patients and may occur anywhere in the mouth.

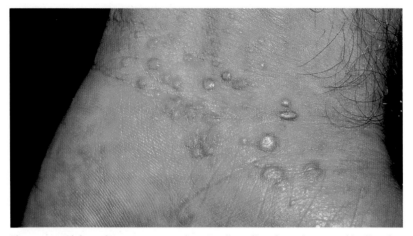

Figure 544. Lichen planus appears to be a T-cell-mediated autoimmune skin disorder. Patients with chronic liver disease (e.g. primary biliary cirrhosis, chronic active hepatitis) have twice the risk of developing lichen planus compared with the general population. Some of these patients are infected with hepatitis B and some with hepatitis C. Purple, polygonal, flat-topped papules, often on the inner wrists, penis, periorbital area, soles, and trunk, occur. A white, lace-like appearance of the surface (Wickham's striae) is characteristic.

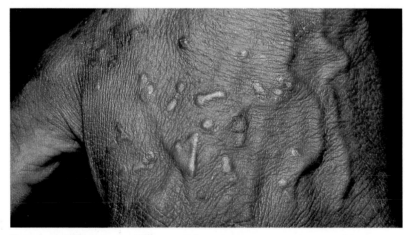

Figure 545. Lichen planus, Köbner.   Lichen planus may occur in areas of trauma. This manual laborer developed several linear lesions on the back of the hands. Note the unique violaceous color that is virtually pathognomonic of lichen planus.

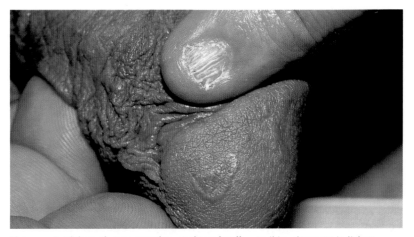

Figure 546. Lichen planus, annular, penis and nail.   Nail involvement in lichen planus may take many forms, including longitudinal ridging, thinning, onycholysis, and pterygium formation. Pterygium is a term used to describe adhesion of the proximal nail plate to the matrix, which may cause significant thinning or absence of the nail. Annular lichen planus, as shown here on the penis, has a predilection for the male genitalia. Lichen planus of the penis may also present as purple papules covered by lace-like Wickham's striae.

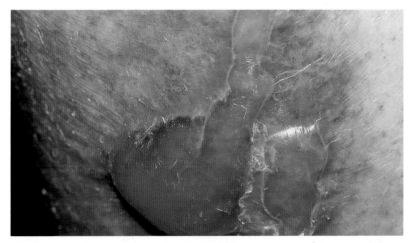

Figure 547. Lichen planus, bullous.   On occasion, the lesions of lichen planus may develop blisters. The blister is a subepidermal bulla showing degeneration of the epidermal basal layer and other features of lichen planus. Bullous lichen planus must be distinguished from lichen planus pemphigoides (LPP) in which the patient with LP develops bullous pemphigoid as well. In LPP, bullae occur apart from the lesions of LP.

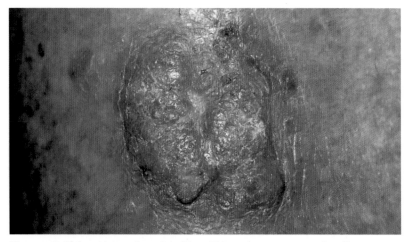

Figure 548. Lichen planus, hypertrophic.   Lichen planus may occasionally present as hyperkeratotic nodules or plaques, especially on the legs.

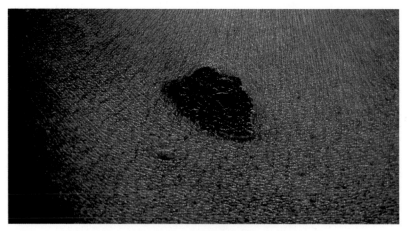

Figure 549. Lichen planus, annular, hyperpigmented.   In lichen planus, there is a tremendous attack on the basal layer of the epidermis. Significant deposition of pigment in the dermis may result. This slowly expanding annular lesion of lichen planus is leaving post-inflammatory hyperpigmentation in its wake.

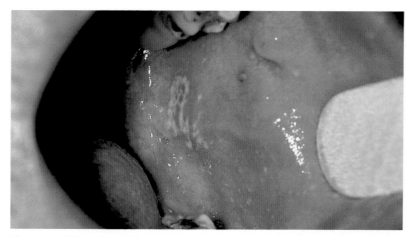

Figure 550. Lichen planus, buccal mucosa. A white, reticulated, lace-like lesion on the buccal mucosa, often bilateral, occurs in lichen planus. This mucosal change is so characteristic of lichen planus that it should be looked for to confirm the diagnosis of lichen planus in atypical cases. Lesions may occur on the tongue and lips as well. It usually is asymptomatic, requiring no treatment.

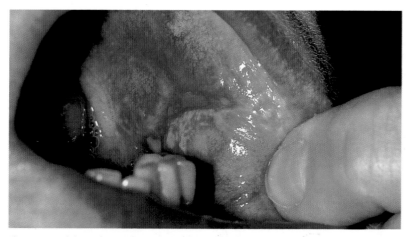

Figure 551. Lichen planus, buccal mucosa, erosive. Oral lichen planus may occasionally erode the mucosa, leading to painful ulcerations. In women, similar changes on the vulvar mucosa may occur. Painful lesions and adhesions can hinder or even prevent intercourse. Rarely, squamous cell carcinoma can arise in either oral or vulvar lichen planus.

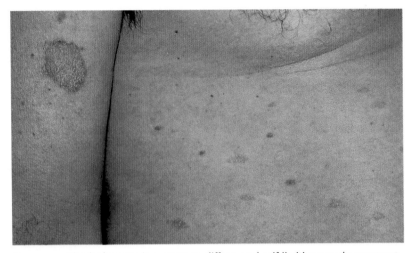

Figure 552. Pityriasis rosea is a common, diffuse, and self-limiting papulosquamous eruption that tends to affect teenagers and young adults. A larger 'herald' patch which predates the more diffuse eruption by 1–3 weeks usually occurs and is shown here on the right arm. Scattered on the trunk are the multiple, oval, red, reasonably well-defined, 1–2 cm plaques with scale. Without the herald patch or other classic features, a rapid plasma reagin should be obtained to rule out secondary syphilis. The rash usually appears over 3 weeks, persists for 3 weeks, and goes away over 3 weeks, although a variant, called chronic pityriasis rosea, may persist.

Figure 553. Pityriasis rosea, incipient. The lesions of pityriasis rosea begin as small erythematous papules, as shown here. The correct diagnosis is rarely made at this stage, unless the herald patch is present. If a patient presents early with only the herald patch, the physician may incorrectly diagnose ringworm, psoriasis, or eczema.

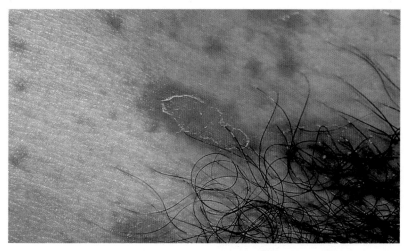

Figure 554. Pityriasis rosea, collarette. The classic, fully developed lesion of pityriasis rosea possesses a peripheral collarette of scale.

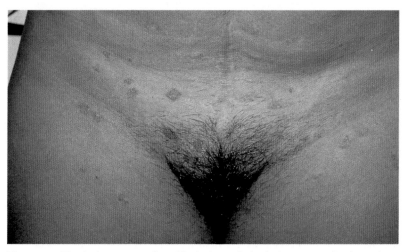

Figure 555. Pityriasis rosea, groin. The lesions of pityriasis rosea prefer the groin and axilla. Occasionally, patients may present with lesions only in these areas. Pityriasis rosea does not like the sun and, in fact, increased sun exposure is one form of treatment.

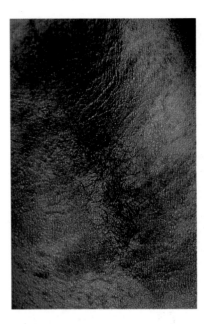

Figure 556. Pityriasis rosea, axilla.
The axilla is another classic site for pityriasis rosea. Lesions may be confluent, as shown here. In the dark-skinned patient, a violaceous hue may be present.

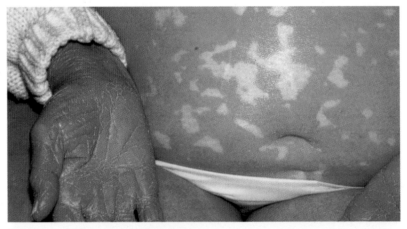

Figure 557. Pityriasis rubra pilaris is a rare chronic papulosquamous disease that is characterized by diffuse erythema about islands of sparing (normal skin) and diffuse hyperkeratosis of the palms and soles. Dramatic follicular plugging may occur on the dorsa of the hands and fingers, like a nutmeg grater. Nail pits are usually absent (compared with psoriasis). The redness and scale of pityriasis rubra pilaris often begin on the scalp and progress downward. Note the prominent islands of sparing on the abdomen in this patient.

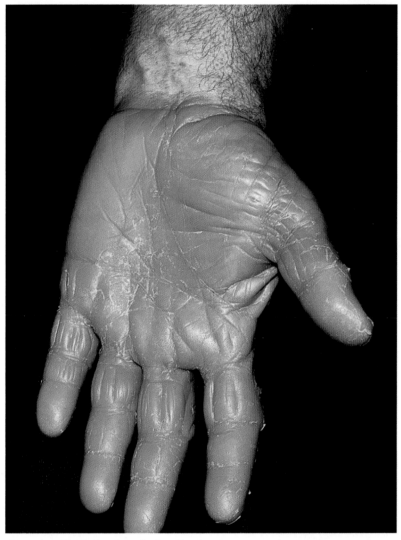

Figure 558. Pityriasis rubra pilaris, palms.

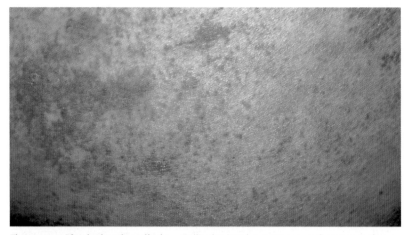

Figure 559. Pityriasis rubra pilaris. Follicular involvement occurs first. Later, these small orangish-red papules merge to form large plaques.

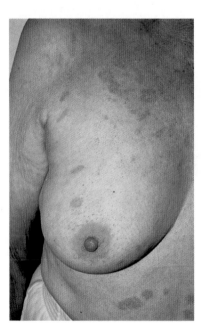

Figure 560. Parapsoriasis, small plaque. The term parapsoriasis refers to chronic papulosquamous lesions in an adult that do not fit the clinical picture of psoriasis. Notably, there is a lack of preference for the elbows, knees, scalp, or nails. Parapsoriasis has been broadly divided into small (<5 cm) and large plaques.

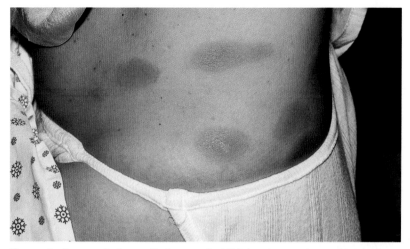

Figure 561. Parapsoriasis, small plaque. Reddish-brown, round to oval, scaly plaques on the trunk that may last years to decades are characteristic of small plaque psoriasis. Elongated or digitate forms occur. Small plaque psoriasis is characteristically non-pruritic. It is generally true that progression to lymphoma does not occur, but periodical biopsy of persistent disease is prudent.

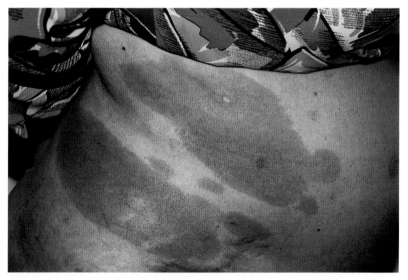

Figure 562. Parapsoriasis, large plaque. Large plaque parapsoriasis is viewed by most as a precursor to cutaneous T-cell lymphoma (CTCL). It may begin insidiously as chronic, fixed, red, scaly lesions. The patient is usually thought to have eczema, psoriasis, or other benign dermatosis and may be treated with topical steroids for years. Histologic examination off topical steroids should be repeated at regular intervals until the diagnosis is confirmed.

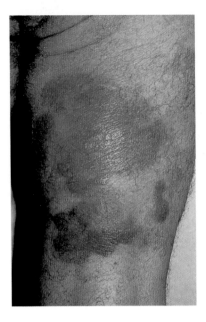

Figure 563. Cutaneous T-cell lymphoma (CTCL) is a slow-growing, peripheral T-cell-derived neoplasm initially confined to the skin. After variable periods, CTCL may progress to involve the blood, lymph nodes, and visceral organs. In CTCL, also known as mycosis fungoides, red, scaly areas develop initially and are followed by infiltrated plaques, figurate lesions, and nodules. The sun-protected areas like the buttocks, thighs, or legs are favored, and lesions are fixed in contrast to eczema.

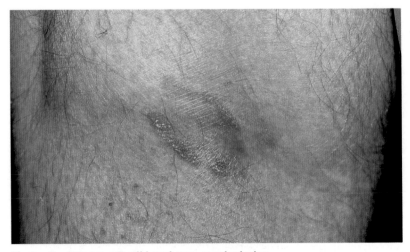

Figure 564. Cutaneous T-cell lymphoma, annular lesion.

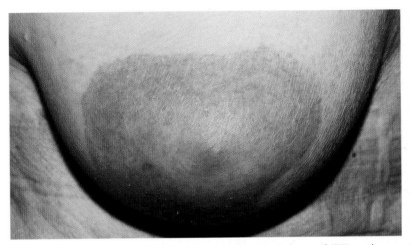

Figure 565. Cutaneous T-cell lymphoma, plaque stage. A plaque of CTCL on the breast.

Figure 566. Cutaneous T-cell lymphoma, poikiloderma. Cutaneous atrophy with prominent telangiectasia is yet another clinical presentation of CTCL.

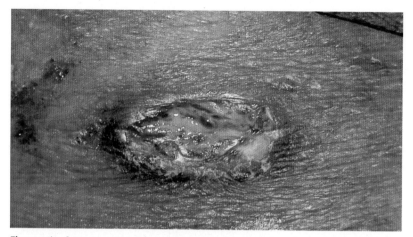

Figure 567. Cutaneous T-cell lymphoma, ulcerative nodule. In the later stages, nodules may develop. They can ulcerate, as shown here. Prognosis is unfavorable if tumors, lymphadenopathy, or skin involvement by infiltrated plaques greater than 10% of body surface area are present.

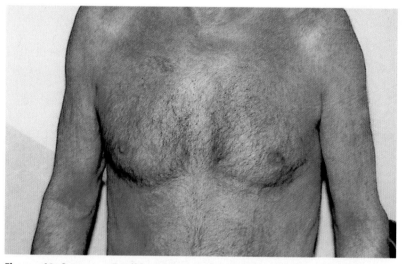

Figure 568. Cutaneous T-cell lymphoma, erythroderma. The adult with diffuse erythroderma may have erythrodermic CTCL. It can develop de novo or as a progression of more typical CTCL. The disease may rapidly progress to involve the lymph nodes and blood or it may progress slowly over years. The Sézary syndrome is the triad of generalized erythroderma, lymphadenopathy, and atypical mononuclear cells in the peripheral blood.

For related disease, see also PLEVA (**Figure 131**).

SKIN MANIFESTATIONS OF SYSTEMIC DISEASE

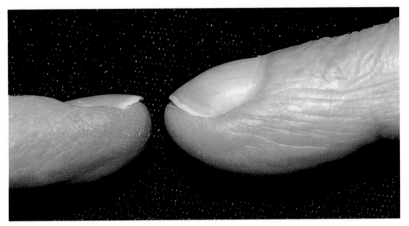

Figure 569. Clubbing. Soft tissue hypertrophy of the distal finger, increased curvature of the nail, and a spongy sensation when the base of the nail is compressed are characteristic. Clubbing may occur as a hereditary, isolated finding, associated with congenital cyanotic heart disease, in thyroid acropachy, or in association with hypertrophic osteoarthropathy (periosteal new bone formation, painful swelling of the distal extremities, arthritis, and malignancy, e.g. bronchogenic carcinoma).

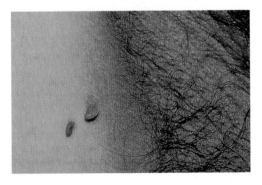

Figure 570. Acanthosis nigricans, neck.
Acanthosis nigricans represents a benign thickening of the skin that may be familial or associated with obesity or diabetes. It is often caused by increased insulin levels. A brown, velvety thickening of the skin on the neck, elbows and dorsa of the hands is seen. Two tags are also present.

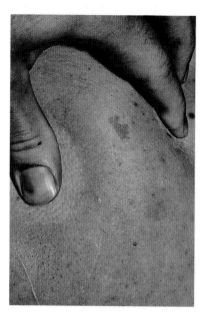

Figure 571. Scleredema diabeticorum.
Firm, non-pitting edema of the upper
back, often in the shape of an inverted
triangle, is characteristic of scleredema
diabeticorum and is common in middle-
aged, obese patients with long-standing
diabetes. This change is usually better
felt than seen.

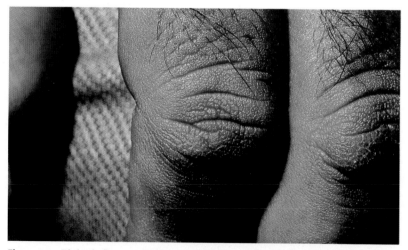

Figure 572. Diabetic finger pebbles. A papillomatous thickening of the skin
overlying the knuckles in diabetic patients has been called diabetic finger pebbles.

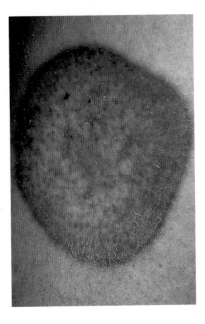

Figure 573. Necrobiosis lipoidica.
Necrobiosis lipoidica diabeticorum is an idiopathic granulomatous skin disorder typically associated with diabetes. Well-demarcated, yellow–red plaques, with epidermal atrophy, on the shins of a diabetic patient, are characteristic. Initially, a red plaque forms. As it spreads, the center becomes depressed and yellow with telangiectasias. Lesions may occur elsewhere and may be unassociated with diabetes.

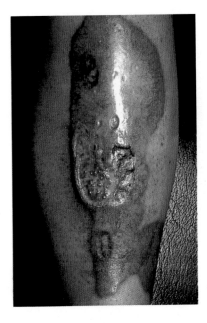

Figure 574. Necrobiosis lipoidica, late, ulcerative. Ulceration is not uncommon in well-developed lesions. (Courtesy of Michael O Murphy, MD.)

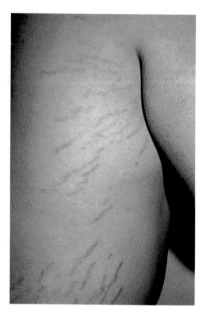

Figure 575. Striae distensae.
Striae are common during adolescence, rapid weight gain, and during pregnancy. They may also follow potent topical steroid use and Cushing's disease. Initially, they are red/purple and eventually fade to leave thin, silvery scars.

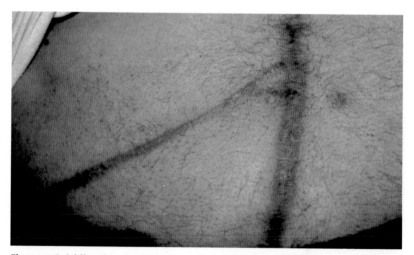

Figure 576. Addisonian pigmentation. Darker pigmentation of photoexposed skin, the nipples and areola, scars (as shown here), the oral mucosa, the periorbital and the anogenital areas may occur in patients with adrenocortical insufficiency or Addison's disease.

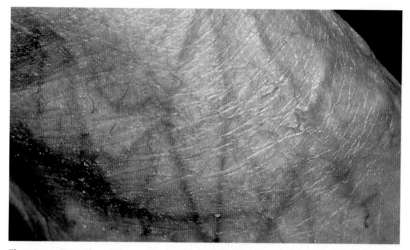

Figure 577. Hypothyroidism. Dry, coarse, cool skin may occasionally be secondary to hypothyroidism. Other cutaneous findings include alopecia of the lateral eyebrows, non-pitting edema, and a diffuse, non-scarring alopecia.

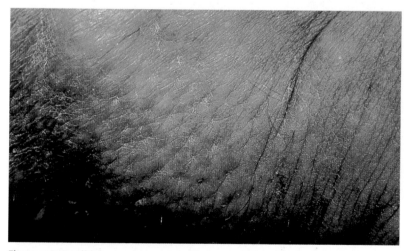

Figure 578. Pretibial myxedema, peau d'orange. Skin-colored or red–brown plaques of the pretibial area of a hyperthyroid patient are characteristic. Various clinical forms have been described, including non-pitting edema (most common), the plaque form, the nodular form, and the elephantiasic form (**Figure 579**). The surface often takes on the appearance of an orange, so-called peau d'orange, as shown here. Almost all patients have high levels of thyroid-stimulating antibodies. The vast majority of patients also have ophthalmopathy, which may be severe, to the point of requiring decompressive surgery.

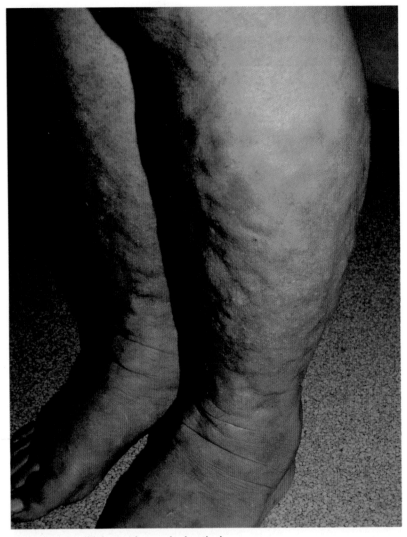

Figure 579. Pretibial myxedema, elephantiasic.

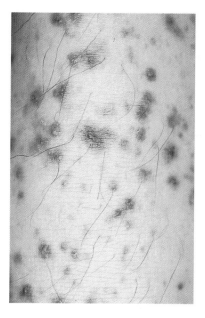

Figure 580. Scurvy. Perifollicular hemorrhage, corkscrew hairs on the legs, easy bleeding, and hypertrophy of the gums, purpura, and epistaxis all occur in scurvy, a deficiency of vitamin C. Patients whose diets may be deficient enough to develop scurvy include elderly, poor, mentally ill, or alcoholic individuals. (Courtesy of Eliot Mostow, MD.)

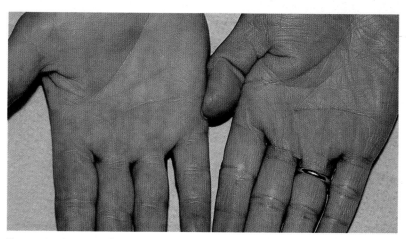

Figure 581. Carotenemia. A diffuse orangish discoloration of the palms in a patient who eats large quantities of carrots occurs in carotenemia. In contrast to jaundice, the eyes are not icteric.

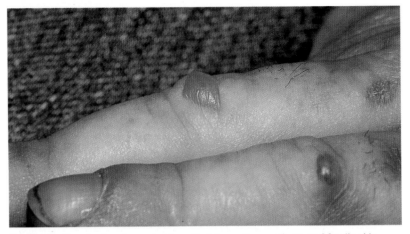

Figure 582. Porphyria cutanea tarda.   Vesicles, milia, erosions, and fragile skin occur symmetrically on the dorsa of the hands in porphyria cutanea tarda. Both an autosomal dominant inherited and an acquired type have been described. For both types, uroporphyrinogen decarboxylase functional activity is low and a history of exposure to alcohol, estrogens, or a liver toxic agent may be found. Hepatitis C virus infection may be found in acquired porphyria cutanea tarda.

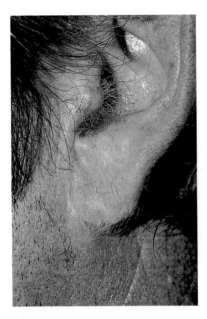

Figure 583. Porphyria cutanea tarda, hypertrichosis.   Look for hypertrichosis along the forehead and on the ears, as shown here.

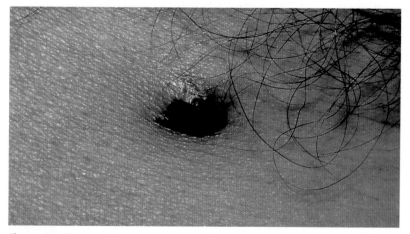

Figure 584. Metastatic lung cancer. Unexplained skin nodules, non-healing ulcers, or persistent indurated erythema may all be manifestations of cutaneous metastatic disease. The principal sites for cutaneous metastasis are the scalp, chest, and abdomen. These lesions may represent a direct extension or hematogenous spread. The most common solid tumors to metastasize to the skin are cancers of the breast and colon and melanoma.

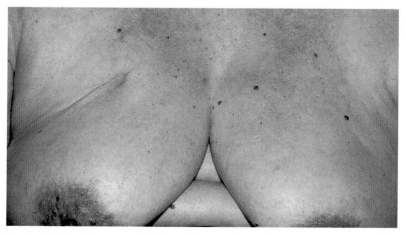

Figure 585. Breast cancer. Nipple or skin retraction or breast asymmetry may develop with breast cancer. A subcutaneous nodule or induration may occur. Skin retraction is seen on the upper part of this woman's breast.

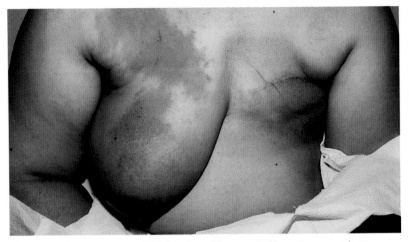

Figure 586. Breast cancer. With lymphangitic spread of breast cancer, a large erythematous plaque may develop which resembles erysipelas, except for its prolonged and relatively static state.

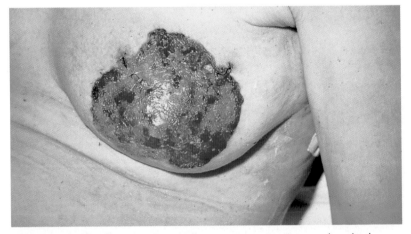

Figure 587. Paget's disease. Paget's disease represents cutaneous invasion by an underlying ductal carcinoma. A chronic, slowly enlarging, sharply demarcated, red, scaly lesion of the nipple and/or breast occurs. There may be ulceration, infiltration, or an underlying, palpable mass. Often, however, the mammogram is normal and no palpable mass is found. The condition is typically mistaken for eczema and treated with topical steroids for years. (Courtesy of Gary Cole, MD.)

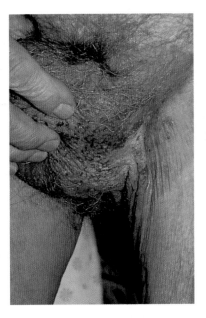

Figure 588. Extramammary Paget's disease presents in an older adult as a slowly expanding, exudative, eczematous or red plaque in the groin, perianal area, or axilla. Each lesion falls into one of three categories: (i) unassociated with an underlying malignancy, presumably representing in-situ malignant transformation of the intraepidermal component of the sweat duct, (ii) epidermotropic spread from an adjacent apocrine or eccrine gland carcinoma, or (iii) epidermotropic spread or metastasis from an underlying cancer (e.g. bladder, rectum, urethra, cervix, or breast).

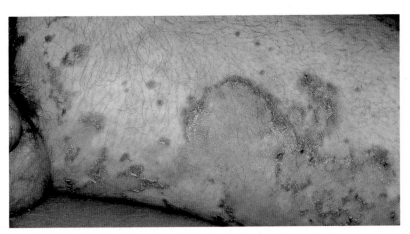

Figure 589. Necrolytic migratory erythema is most commonly a cutaneous manifestation of a glucagon-secreting, alpha-cell tumor of the pancreas, although some patients may have necrolytic migratory erythema without a glucagonoma. An annular, erosive, or bullous eruption develops periorally and in the groin. Weight loss, anemia, diabetes mellitus, and glossitis may occur.

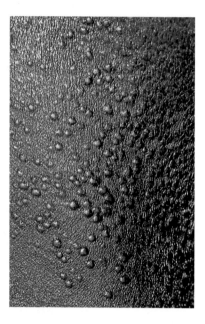

Figure 590. Lichen myxedematosis.
Cutaneous mucin deposition may occur in association with a paraprotein usually of the IgG-lambda type. When multiple cutaneous papules occur, the term lichen myxedematosis is used (also papular mucinosis). When confluent with underlying induration, the term scleromyxedema is used. Diffuse deposition of mucin may occur internally, although life expectancy is usually not affected. Gastrointestinal involvement is most common, manifested for example by dysphagia or abnormal upper GI series. Other systemic manifestations include dyspnea on exertion, hypogonadism, hypothyroidism, diabetes mellitus, and proximal muscle weakness. In lichen myxedematosis, innumerable uniform, 2–3 mm, skin-colored papules along the arms, neck, and face are seen.

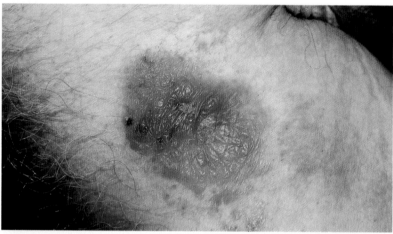

Figure 591. Nodular amyloid represents a localized accumulation of amyloid derived from the degradation of immunoglobulin light chains. Initially, a population of plasma cells in the skin secrete immunoglobulin light chains. These are phagocytosed by macrophages and processed, resulting in the deposition of insoluble amyloid fibrils. Cutaneous nodules representing deposits of amyloid may occur alone or in association with systemic amyloid. In this context, the term nodular amyloid refers to cutaneous lesions in the absence of systemic disease. A work-up should be done to exclude both systemic amyloid and multiple myeloma. Nodular amyloidosis progresses to systemic amyloidosis in 5–10% of cases. Clinically, one sees single or multiple waxy plaques or nodules in an older adult. The consistency of the lesion may be rubbery, firm, waxlike, or anetodermic.

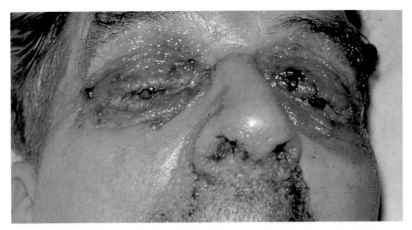

Figure 592. Systemic amyloidosis. Periorbital waxy papules and nodules, along with petechiae and purpura after the slightest trauma (pinch purpura) are characteristic of this infiltrative disease. Post-proctoscopic periorbital purpura is a classic but uncommon presentation. A paraprotein is found in the majority, and approximately one-third of patients have an associated myeloma. (Courtesy of Department of Dermatology, University of California, San Diego.)

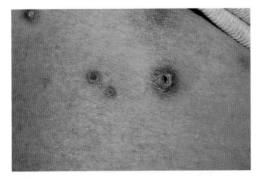

Figure 593. Perforating disorder of dialysis. Hyperkeratotic papules on the thighs of a patient with renal failure (usually from diabetes mellitus) and on dialysis are characteristic. Material from the dermis is being extruded through the central hyperkeratotic core of each papule. Lesions may be very pruritic, and a component of prurigo nodularis may be present.

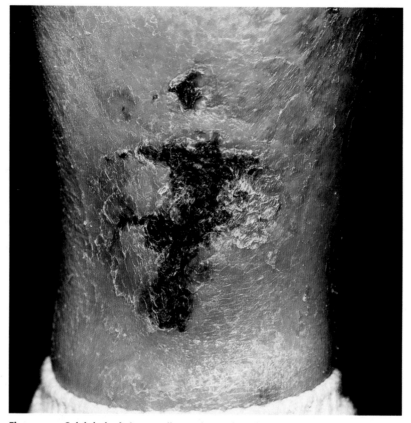

Figure 594. Calciphylaxis is a small vessel vasculopathy associated with soft tissue calcification that occurs predominantly in individuals with renal failure on dialysis. It causes ischemia and necrosis of skin, subcutaneous fat, visceral organs, and skeletal muscle. The syndrome causes significant morbidity in the form of infection, organ failure, and pain. Mortality is high. Painful mottling of the skin, resembling livedo reticularis, is characteristic of the initial lesion. Later, these areas become indurated, echymotic plaques that enlarge and develop central necrosis and ulceration. Distal gangrene and autoamputation of multiple digits are common. Extensive calcification of blood vessels may be seen histologically and on radiographs.

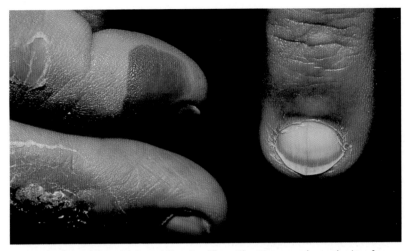

Figure 595. Pseudoporphyria and Terry's nails. The term pseudoporphyria refers to vesicles and fragility on the dorsa of the hands resulting from exposure to both a weak sensitizer (e.g. a sulfonamide, dapsone, furosemide, nalidixic acid, naproxen, pyridoxone, fluoroquinolone antibiotics, or tetracycline) and significant ultraviolet light (e.g. from the sun or a tanning bed). The clinical presentation is nearly identical to porphyria cutanea tarda (thus pseudoporphyria). However, urine porphyrin levels are normal, and hypertrichosis is absent. Patients with renal failure, and especially those on dialysis, are at increased risk for developing this condition. Terry's nails are also present in this patient (white nail with distal pink rim).

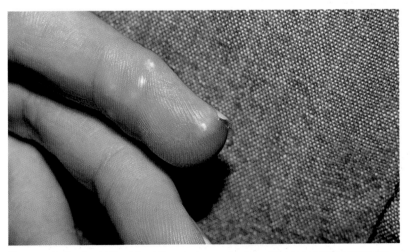

Figure 596. Gout. Yellowish-white papules on the fingertips may rarely occur as a manifestation of gout. Whitish or flesh-colored papulonodules may also occur on the rim of the ears, elbows, and over the knuckles. These tophi are deposits of monosodium urate crystals. Special fixation of the skin biopsy is needed so as not to dissolve the urate crystals.

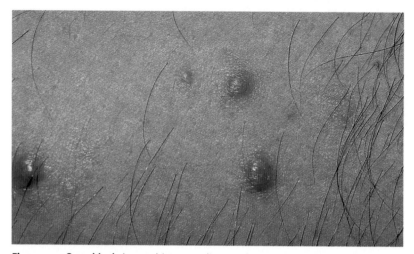

Figure 597. Sarcoidosis is a multi-system disease characterized by non-caseating granulomas. It affects many organ systems, including the skin, lungs, eyes, and bone. Its cause is unknown. Sarcoidosis is more common in dark-skinned patients. It may manifest itself in the skin in many ways, including papules (**Figure 597**, top), plaques (**Figure 598**), nodules, annular lesions, ulcers, ichthyosis, scar infiltration, erythroderma, lupus pernio (**Figure 599**), ungual lesions, hypopigmented plaques (**Figure 600**), and erythema nodosum. Ocular (uveitis, iris nodules, conjunctivitis), pulmonary, musculoskeletal (polyarthritis, bone cysts), and lymph node involvement are common. Granulomas may be found in the kidneys, heart and elsewhere.

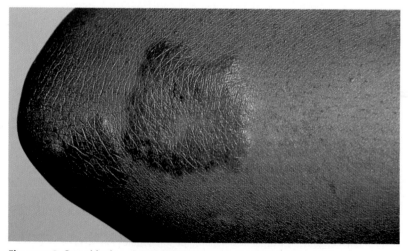

Figure 598. Sarcoidosis.   Dermal plaques without epidermal change in an African-American patient are very characteristic of sarcoidosis.

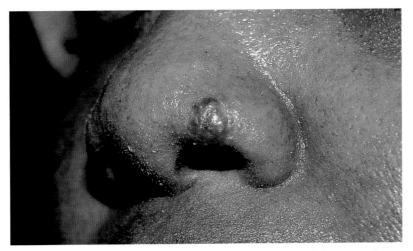

Figure 599. Sarcoidosis, lupus pernio.   Red, smooth papules and plaques on the nose and other acral areas, such as the ears, fingers, and toes, occur in lupus pernio, a subtype of sarcoidosis. Bone cysts of the fingers may be associated.

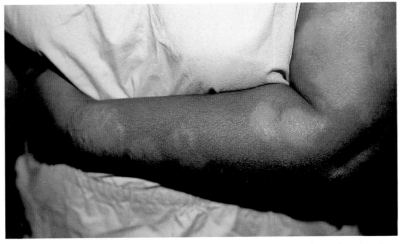

Figure 600. Sarcoidosis, hypopigmented.   The skin may become hypopigmented over plaques of sarcoidosis.

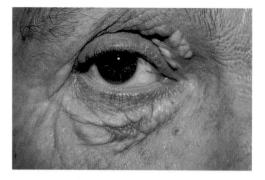

Figure 601. Xanthelasma. Soft, yellow plaques on the upper, inner eyelids are characteristic of xanthelasma. They may occur as an isolated finding or in association with a hyperlipidemia. In more severe cases, lesions may also occur infra-orbitally as shown here.

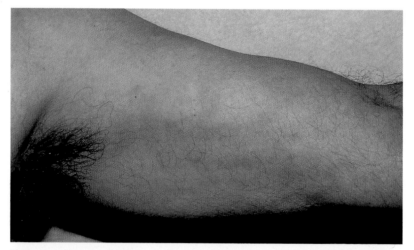

Figure 602. Plane xanthoma. Large yellow patches or very slightly elevated yellow plaques are characteristic and are illustrated here on the arm of this patient with myeloma. Plane xanthomas may be subdivided into three groups: (i) associated with other xanthomas and part of a familial hyperlipidemia or secondary to liver disease, usually biliary cirrhosis, (ii) associated with a paraprotein and elevated lipids, or (iii) associated with a paraprotein but no elevation in the lipids. In groups (ii) and (iii), the paraprotein seems to interfere with lipid metabolism and may cause a lipoprotein–paraprotein complex with either elevation of the lipids or increase in their phagocytosis by macrophages.

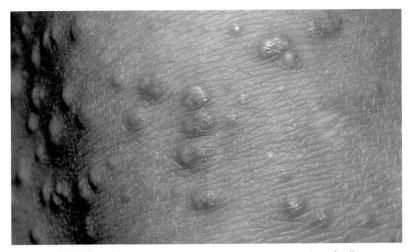

Figure 603. Eruptive xanthoma. A widespread, symmetric eruption of yellow papules with preference for the knees, elbows, and buttocks occurs in eruptive xanthoma. Conditions that predispose to the eruption include diabetes mellitus, chronic renal failure, nephrotic syndrome, hypothyroidism, alcohol ingestion, underlying hypertriglyceridemia, and certain drugs (e.g. isotretinoin).

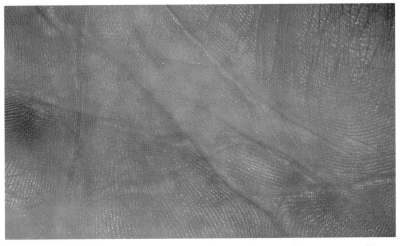

Figure 604. Xanthoma palmare is a type of plane xanthoma and presents as yellow palmar creases. It usually occurs in type III (broad beta) hyperlipidemia. (Courtesy of Stephen H Ducatman, MD.)

SUN DAMAGE/NON-MELANOMA SKIN CANCERS

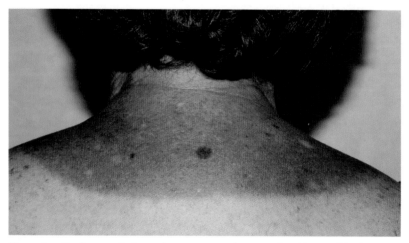

Figure 605. Sunburn. Prolonged sun exposure damages the skin, resulting in inflammation, erythema, and tenderness—also known as 'sunburn'. Blisters may form. Later, desquamation occurs. Sunburns before the age of 20 are associated with more melanocytic and atypical melanocytic nevi, and melanoma.

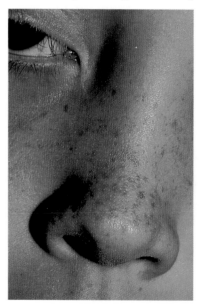

Figure 606. Freckles/ephelides. Light tan or brown macules scattered on the face or nose of a light-skinned, red-haired patient are characteristic. The nose is preferentially affected as it receives sunlight more directly. The health care provider should encourage the parents of affected children to apply sunscreen.

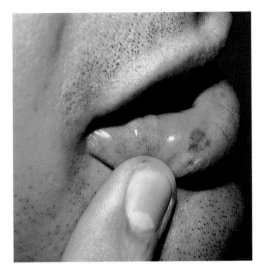

Figure 607. Labial melanotic macule.
A pigmented macule on the lower lip, usually in the middle third, is seen. This large 'freckle' or lentigo is caused by chronic sun exposure. Teenagers and young adults are most commonly affected.

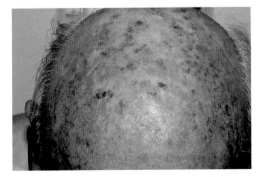

Figure 608. Photodamaged skin, scalp. Aged skin without sun damage is thin and lacking in subcutaneous fat. Chronic photodamage adds mottled pigmentation, solar elastosis, additional wrinkling, and, to the susceptible, actinic keratoses, basal cell and squamous cell carcinomas. Hats are an essential part of protection, especially as the hair thins.

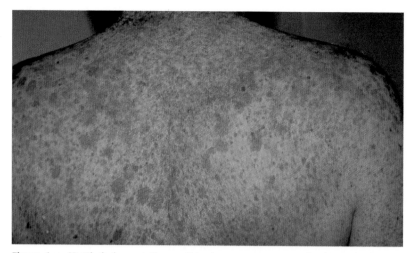

Figure 609. Mottled pigmentation.   Chronic sun exposure may lead to multiple brown macules or lentigines. Hypopigmentation and telangiectases may also develop. Melanomas of course may also occur, and so all pigmented lesions should be evaluated by the ABCD criteria (see **Figure 489**), and, if two are present, a biopsy should be performed.

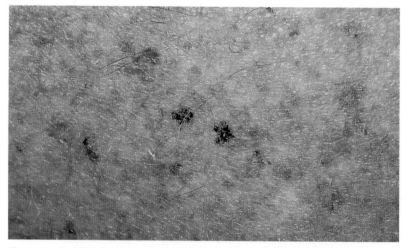

Figure 610. Lentigo, ink dot.   An especially dark, irregularly pigmented macule like an ink drop may occur on the upper back and is completely benign.

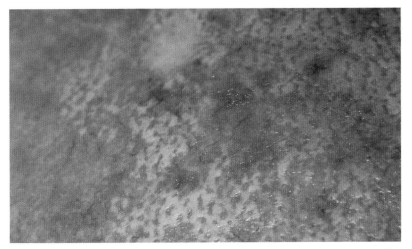

Figure 611. Solar elastosis.   A reticulate pattern of yellow papules is seen below the thinned skin. The forehead of men with a receding hairline is most commonly affected.

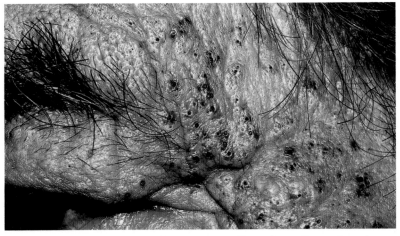

Figure 612. Favre–Racouchot syndrome.   Cysts, milia, and comedones about the lateral eyes and cheeks in a middle-aged to elderly patient with a significant history of sun exposure are characteristic. Note the tremendous number of comedones about the eyes in this patient.

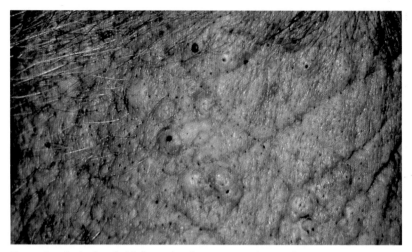

Figure 613. Cutis rhomboidalis nuchae/Favre–Racouchot syndrome. Diagonal furrows that criss-cross the nape, forming rhomboids in an older patient after much sun exposure, are characteristic of cutis rhomboidalis nuchae. Cysts and comedones of Favre–Racouchot syndrome are also seen.

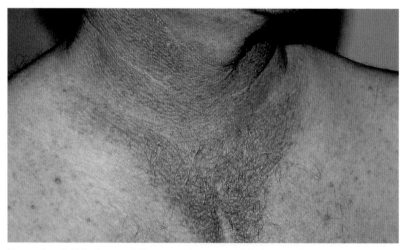

Figure 614. Poikiloderma of Civatte. The term poikiloderma refers to the combination of mottled pigmentation, telangiectasia, and cutaneous atrophy. It may occur about the neck as a result of chronic sun exposure.

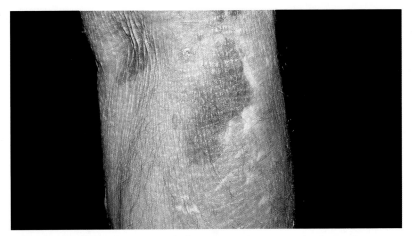

Figure 615. Age-related purpura.   Red–purple patches, 1–4 cm in size, on the exterior forearms or dorsa of the hands in the older photodamaged arm are characteristic of age-related purpura. These bruises are precipitated by the slightest trauma. Old age and chronic steroid use, especially intramuscularly, predispose to these lesions. Other terms that have been used include senile purpura and solar purpura.

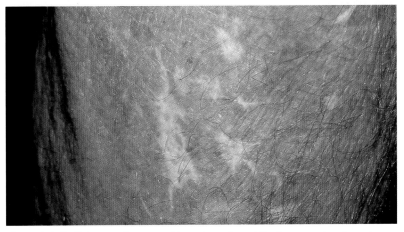

Figure 616. Stellate pseudoscars.   These irregular, white, linear or star-shaped lesions occur on the sun-exposed forearms of older people. Chronic steroid use may predispose the patient to their formation.

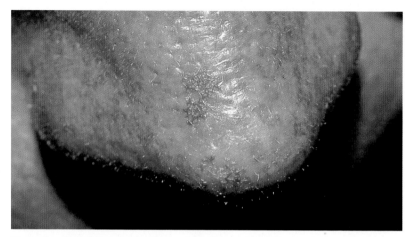

Figure 617. Actinic keratosis, nose. A fixed, hyperkeratotic, or scaly papule on the face, arms, or hands of an adult is characteristic of this premalignant, UV-induced condition. The patient often complains of a burning or itching sensation. The scaly papule periodically falls off—often just before the doctor's appointment! These lesions are often better felt than seen, and thus the physician should not be afraid to touch the patient in order to find them.

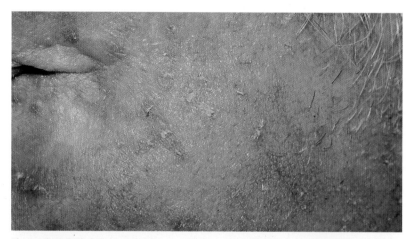

Figure 618. Actinic keratosis, face, multiple. Multiple actinic keratoses are seen on this man's left cheek and temple. The presence of multiple actinic keratoses is one of the strongest predictors of future basal cell carcinoma (BCC) or squamous cell carcinoma (SCC). Regular sunscreen use, sun avoidance, and a low fat diet reduce their numbers.

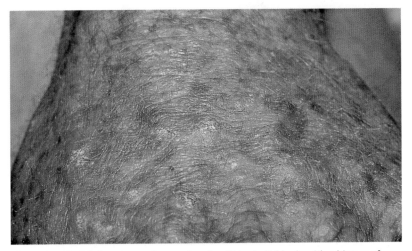

Figure 619. Actinic keratoses, dorsum hand.   Older individuals with a history of chronic sun exposure may develop hyperkeratotic papules or scaly areas on the dorsa of the hands. The majority represent hypertrophic actinic keratoses (as shown here). The differential diagnosis for large lesions would include a SCC and, if rapidly growing, a keratoacanthoma. Basal cell carcinoma, for some reason, is rare on the dorsa of the hands.

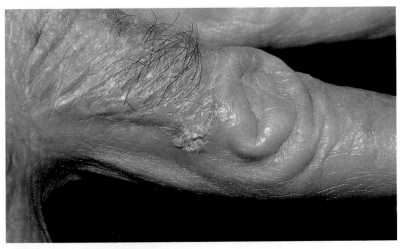

Figure 620. Actinic keratosis, finger.   The dorsa of the fingers should not be forgotten during a cutaneous examination.

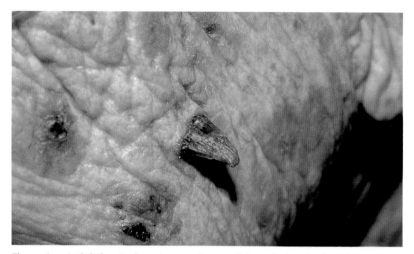

Figure 621. Actinic keratosis, cutaneous horn. This conical projection of compact hyperkeratosis usually overlies an actinic keratosis, although a SCC, seborrheic keratosis, or verruca may be found.

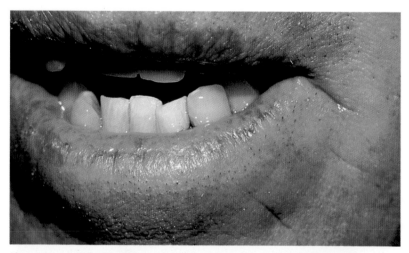

Figure 622. Actinic cheilitis. A fixed hyperkeratotic papule or diffuse scale on the lower lip is characteristic of actinic cheilitis, which is a common premalignant condition occurring after years of sun exposure. Palpation for induration or thickening that might signal an underlying squamous cell carcinoma is critically important.

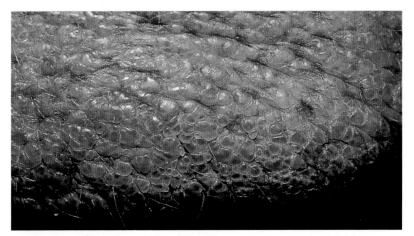

Figure 623. Colloid milia. This condition is the end result of decades of sun exposure. Firm papules on the dorsa of the hands, arms (as shown here), forehead, or cheeks in an older patient are characteristic.

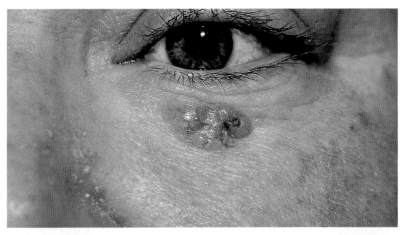

Figure 624. Basal cell carcinoma, nodular. The basal cell carcinoma is the most common type of skin cancer and it arises from the basal cell layer of the epidermis. Risk factors include sunbed use, radiotherapy, a family history of skin cancers, type I skin, a tendency to freckle in childhood, and Irish, Scottish, Scandinavian, or German heritage. The BCC can take on many appearances. A slowly expanding pearly papule with telangiectasias on the face of an older person is classic. Routine follow-up should occur for any patient with BCC, as approximately 40% will develop a second BCC within 5 years.

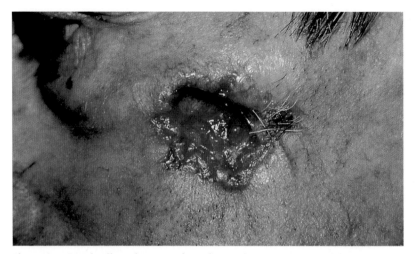

Figure 625. Basal cell carcinoma, rodent ulcer. If untreated, the nodule expands and undergoes central ulceration. The edge is often described as having a rolled border. The term rodent ulcer is sometimes used, as if a rat had gnawed a hole in the skin. BCC rarely metastasizes. When it does, the patient usually has a very large lesion (e.g. >10 cm) that has been present for many years.

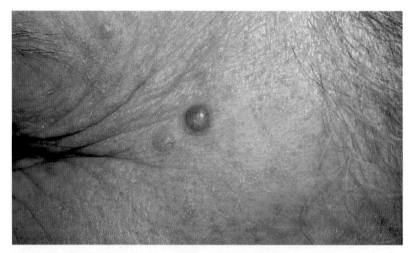

Figure 626. Basal cell carcinoma, nodular. The possibility of a BCC should be considered with any slowly growing papule or nodule on the face of a fair-skinned adult. It may be clinically impossible to distinguish a flesh-colored nevus from a BCC. The reddish papule with telangiectasia in the center of the photograph is a BCC. The smaller papule to the left and below is a benign nevus.

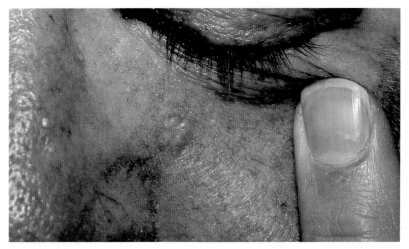

Figure 627. Basal cell carcinoma, morpheaform. The morpheaform or fibrosing BCC often has a whitish or yellowish hue. It is typically flat or even depressed, and the margins are ill-defined.

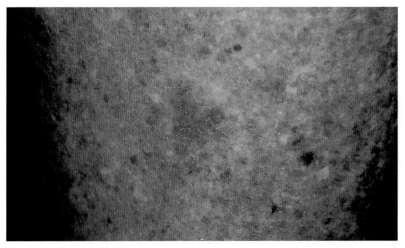

Figure 628. Superficial basal cell carcinoma. This variant of BCC usually presents as a slowly enlarging, red, scaly area on the back of an older adult with significant sun exposure. Ulceration is unusual. The process is limited to the superficial layers of the skin.

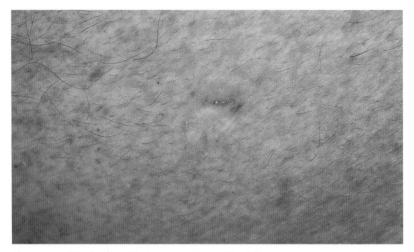

Figure 629. Basal cell carcinoma, recurrent. The follow-up examination of any patient with a history of a BCC should include an examination with palpation of the scar for recurrence. Surface changes including redness, scale, or crust should arouse suspicion, as should a new dermal papule. In the figure, redness and slight scale just superior to the whitish scar represents a recurrence of a superficial BCC which had previously undergone electrodesiccation and curettage.

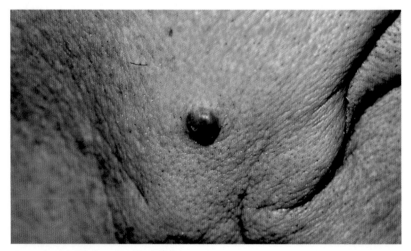

Figure 630. Cystic basal cell carcinoma. A blue–purple, dermal nodule is typical of this uncommon variant of BCC. The cyst is formed by necrosis and degeneration of the center of a solid (nodular) BCC.

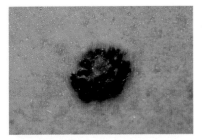

Figure 631. Pigmented basal cell in a Filipino man. This variant is similar to the nodular BCC except for the abundant pigment. Such lesions may mimic melanoma. Dark-skinned patients, but not black patients, are at greatest risk. (See also **Figure 486**.)

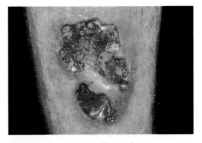

Figure 632. Basal cell carcinoma mimicking chronic stasis ulcer. Occasionally, an ulcer on the leg may represent a BCC or an SCC. Often, such lesions are treated for years as a stasis ulcer. This lesion was treated for 6 years as a stasis ulcer.

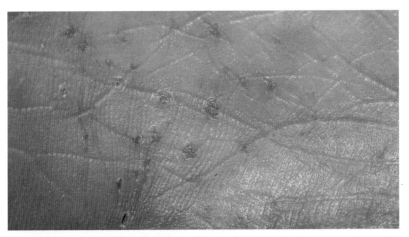

Figure 633. Basal cell nevus syndrome, plantar pits. Basal cell nevus syndrome is an autosomal dominant disease characterized by the presence of multiple basal cell carcinomas, odontogenic keratocysts, and palmoplantar pits. Associated abnormalities involve the CNS (e.g. mental retardation, calcification of the falx cerebri, congenital hydrocephalus–macrocephaly, medulloblastoma, meningioma, cysts), bones (e.g. a characteristic fascies, a marfanoid habitus, fused, bifid, or missing ribs, odontogenic keratocysts of the jaw, vertebral abnormalities), and eyes (e.g. congenital cataracts, glaucoma).

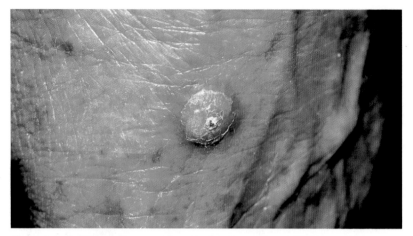

Figure 634. Keratoacanthoma, early. The keratoacanthoma (KA) is a rapidly growing tumor, usually of the sun-exposed skin, that mimics a squamous cell carcinoma. In fact, the distinction between keratoacanthoma and SCC both clinically and histologically is often difficult. The classic KA resolves spontaneously, but lesions may rarely become huge by unrestricted growth. Chronic UV exposure is a predisposing factor, and the patient should be examined for other non-melanoma skin cancers. HPV DNA is found in a small percentage of lesions. A rapidly growing nodule that develops a central keratotic core in the sun-exposed area of an elderly person is characteristic. The hands and arms as well as the head and neck are commonly affected.

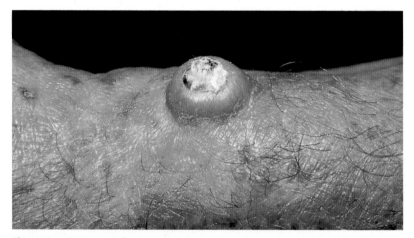

Figure 635. Keratoacanthoma. This figure shows the classic features of a mature lesion. A dome-shaped nodule with a central horn-filled core is seen. Growth to this size usually takes about 2 months.

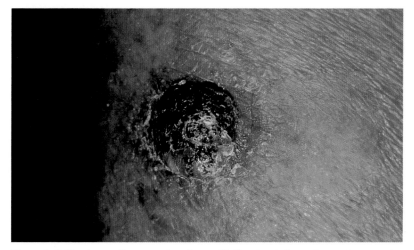

Figure 636. Keratoacanthoma, regressing. If left untreated, most keratoacanthomas regress, usually within 6 months.

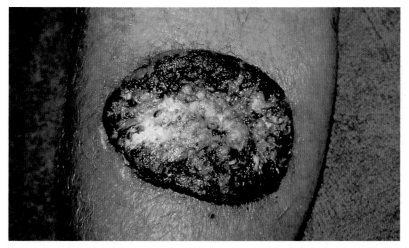

Figure 637. Keratoacanthoma, giant. Although most keratoacanthomas regress if left untreated, a small percentage do not. A progressively enlarging verrucous lesion with central clearing or atrophy is the result. The periphery of the lesion shows typical features of keratoacanthoma, whereas the center may show atrophy and dermal scarring. Diameters of 5–30 cm have been reported.

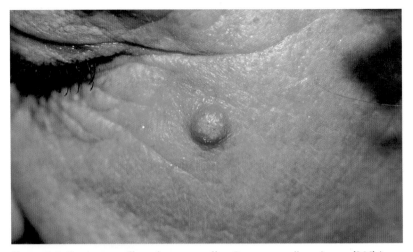

Figure 638. Squamous cell carcinoma, small.   Squamous cell carcinoma (SCC) is the second most common skin cancer. It arises from the squamous cells of the epidermis. Chronic ultraviolet light exposure is the main risk factor, although HPV plays an oncogenic role in some lesions. A hyperkeratotic, enlarging plaque or nodule, usually in a photoexposed area of an older adult, is characteristic. Those on the lip, within scars, and in areas not exposed to the sun must be considered more aggressive, but even small SCCs in sun-exposed areas may metastasize. Those patients at increased risk for SCC have light skin, blonde or red hair, a tendency to burn rather than tan in the sun, and chronic occupational solar exposure.

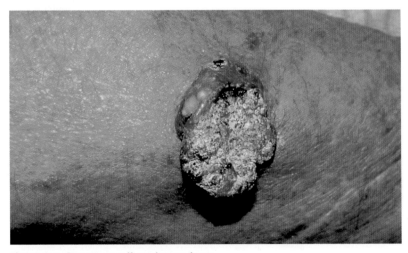

Figure 639. Squamous cell carcinoma, large.

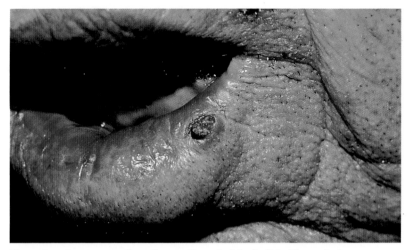

Figure 640. Squamous cell carcinoma, lip.   Actinic cheilitis (**Figure 622**) may progress to invasive SCC. A slowly enlarging, hyperkeratotic papulonodule originating from the vermilion border of the lower lip is characteristic. Squamous cell carcinoma of the lip has a higher incidence of metastasis than does cutaneous SCC.

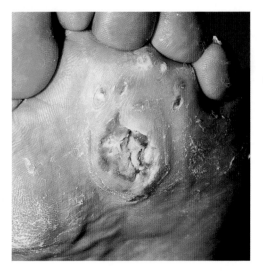

Figure 641. Verrucous carcinoma.   Several low grade squamous cell carcinomas fall under the term verrucous carcinoma. These include oral florid papillomatosis (mouth), Buscke Lowenstein tumor (penis), and carcinoma cunniculatum (sole, shown here). The verrucous carcinoma of the sole often resembles a wart. Indeed, some of these lesions may have begun as a wart.

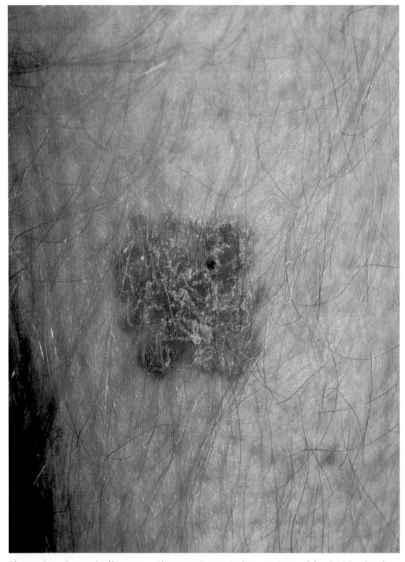

Figure 642. Bowen's disease. The term Bowen's disease is used for SCC in situ that has a characteristic histopathologic picture. Clinically, one finds a slowly enlarging, sharply demarcated, red, scaly plaque. It may occur on sun-exposed or sun-protected sites. Many patients have a history of either BCC or SCC.

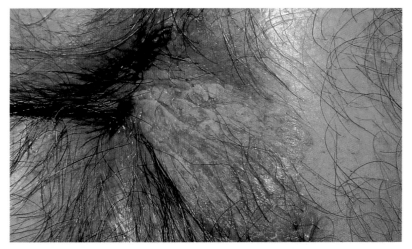

Figure 643. Bowen's disease, perianal.   A well-demarcated, red, scaly, moist plaque in the perianal area that is slow growing over years is characteristic.

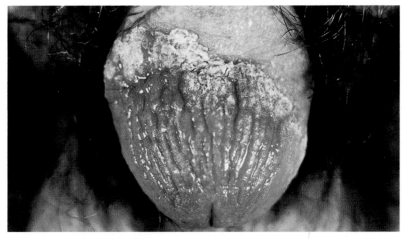

Figure 644. Erythroplasia of Queyrat is a term used to describe squamous cell carcinoma in situ of the penis. An underlying invasive SCC may be found. Several risk factors have been noted, including lack of circumcision in infancy or early childhood, HPV infection, balanitis, and smoking. Other factors may be related, including the chronic presence of smegma (which may be converted to carcinogenic agents by *Mycobacterium smegmatis*), phimosis, PUVA therapy, and the presence of lichen sclerosis. A fixed red, moist patch/plaque on the glans of an uncircumcised elderly man is characteristic. (Courtesy of Michael O Murphy, MD.)

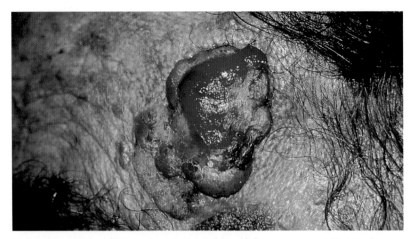

Figure 645. Atypical fibroxanthoma, ulcerative nodule. An atypical fibroxanthoma is a cutaneous tumor akin to a malignant fibrous histiocytoma but less aggressive. It most commonly occurs in an older person on the head and neck, presumably related to chronic sun exposure. A solitary papule that grows to an ulcerated nodule on the head or neck in an older Caucasian person is characteristic. Bleeding and ulceration are common. Metastasis may rarely occur. Immunohistochemical studies are needed to exclude SCC and melanoma.

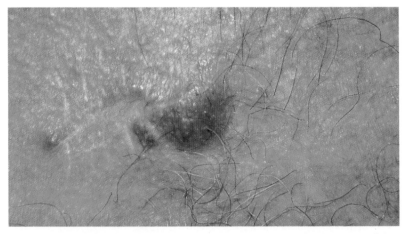

Figure 646. Merkel cell carcinoma is a rare, aggressive neuroendocrine tumor of the skin which arises from Merkel cells or an epithelial precursor cell. It is commonly seen in the elderly on the head, neck, and extremities, with a predisposition for local, regional, and distant spreading. A solitary, red–purple or violaceous, shiny, dome-shaped nodule or plaque on the face, head, or neck of an elderly person is characteristic. Twenty percent occur in the periorbital area. Mortality is high. (Courtesy of Duane Whitaker, MD.)

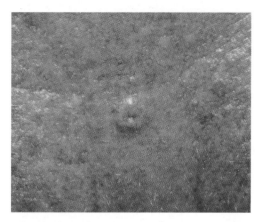

Figure 647. Sebaceous hyperplasia. These 2–4 mm 'yellow donuts' develop on the face with age. Favored sites are the forehead, temples, and cheeks. There is no correlation with sun exposure or solar elastosis.

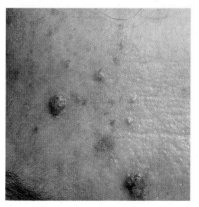

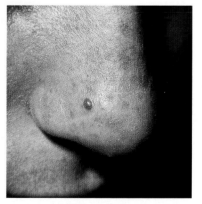

Figure 648. Sebaceous adenoma. In contrast to sebaceous hyperplasia, the presence of even one sebaceous neoplasm should prompt the consideration of Muir–Torre's syndrome. Muir–Torre's syndrome is the association of sebaceous neoplasms (e.g. sebaceous adenoma, sebaceous epithelioma, basal cell epithelioma with sebaceous differentiation, or sebaceous carcinoma) with low grade visceral carcinomas and keratoacanthomas. In the patient pictured, the three yellowish papules on the forehead are sebaceous adenomas.

Figure 649. Fibrous papule. This benign papular lesion is commonly mistaken for a small nevus. Typically, a small (2–4 mm), flesh-colored or red solitary papule occurs on or about the nose.

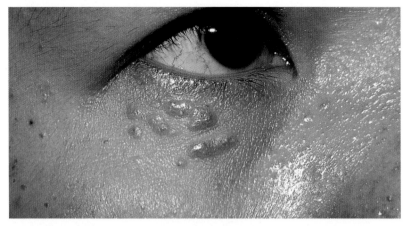

Figure 650. Syringomas, periorbital. These tumorous collections of sweat glands commonly occur infra-orbitally in patients of Asian descent. Rarely, they may be distributed diffusely on the face or body or be present as a solitary lesion.

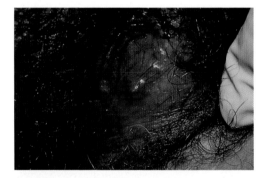

Figure 651. Hidradenoma papilliferum. A solitary dermal papule or nodule in the vulvar or perivulvar area is characteristic of this adnexal tumor of apocrine origin.

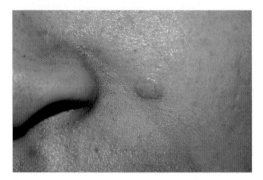

Figure 652. Trichoepithelioma, solitary. This papule, usually located on the face, commonly resembles a nevus or a basal cell carcinoma. A yellowish-white color and a depressed center are distinguishing features.

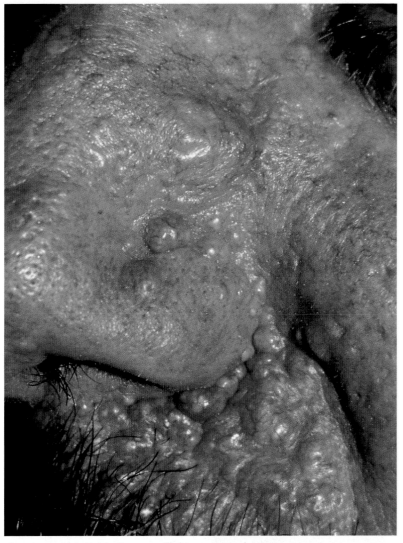

Figure 653. Trichoepithelioma, multiple. As with many adnexal tumors, trichoepitheliomas may occur multiply, inherited as an autosomal dominant trait. Multiple, symmetric, flesh-colored papules occur characteristically along the nasolabial folds and upper lip, with onset in the teens. Lesions on the ear and forehead also occur. Cylindromas of the scalp may be associated.

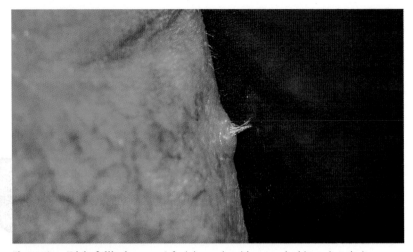

Figure 654. Trichofolliculoma. A facial papule with several white, wispy hairs emanating from the center is characteristic.

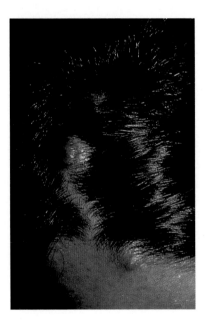

Figure 655. Cylindroma. Cylindromas present as solitary or multiple, firm, dermal nodules on the scalp. When multiple, the condition is often inherited autosomal dominantly and trichoepitheliomas may be associated. (Courtesy of Michael O Murphy, MD.)

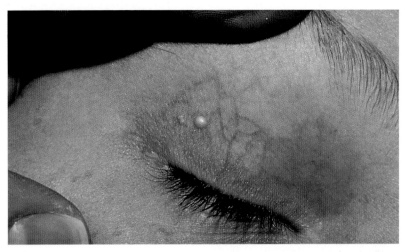

Figure 656. Milia.   A woman will commonly complain about these tiny, facial 'white heads' that just will not 'pop'. In reality, they represent miniature epidermal inclusion cysts.

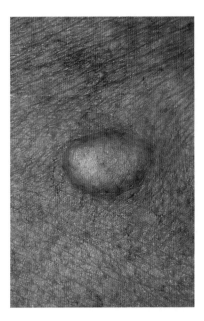

Figure 657. Epidermal inclusion cyst. A dermal nodule, at times with a visible pore, is a common occurrence in adults. Lesions typically occur on the back, neck, and face. When superficial, the nodule may be whitish in color. The lesion grows slowly over time and may periodically drain. The patient commonly complains that the extruded material is foul smelling.

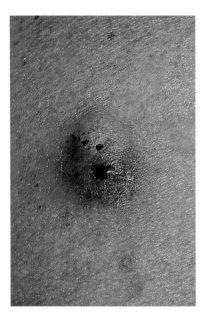

Figure 658. Epidermal inclusion cyst, ruptured.   Occasionally, the cyst wall of an epidermal inclusion cyst ruptures into the dermis, causing an intense inflammatory foreign body response. Swelling, erythema, and pain occur. The inflammation may remain deep and slowly resolve over weeks to a month or it may become fluctuant and drain spontaneously, as shown here.

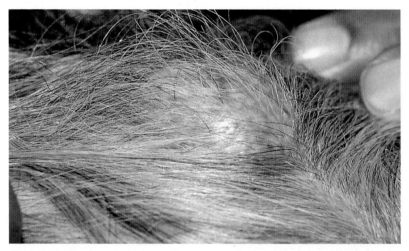

Figure 659. Pilar cyst.   This type of cyst occurs almost exclusively on the scalp. It is firm, round and usually non-tender. When multiple, it may be inherited autosomal dominantly.

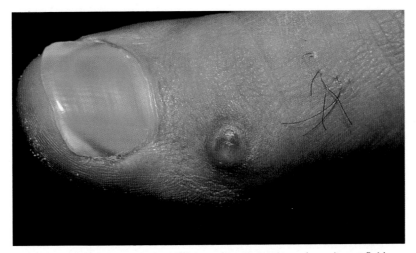

Figure 660. Digital mucous cyst. This pseudocyst contains a clear, viscous fluid representing an abnormal production of ground substance. Why it prefers the area between the distal interphalangeal joint and the nail is unknown. If it impinges on the nail matrix, a groove may form in the nail plate (see **Figure 455**). Hemorrhage into the lesions may occur, turning them blue or black.

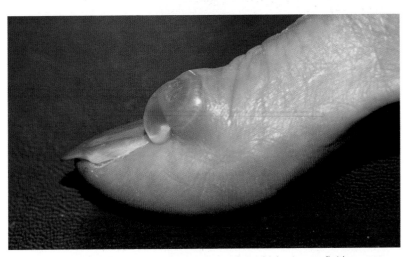

Figure 661. Digital mucous cyst. On rupture, a clear, thick, viscous fluid emanates.

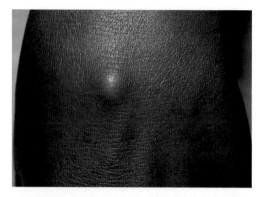

Figure 662. Ganglion cyst. A 1–3 cm subcutaneous nodule overlying the ankle or wrist may represent a ganglion cyst.

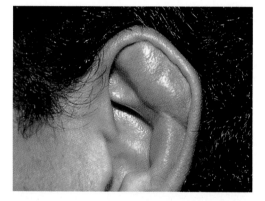

Figure 663. Pseudocyst, ear. A non-tender, firm, cystic lesion of the ear is characteristic. It may be preceded by trauma as occurred in two boys after ear pulling for their birthday. It also may be associated with atopic dermatitis. Drainage yields a thick, viscous fluid.

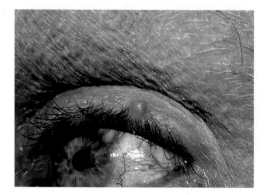

Figure 664. Apocrine hydrocystoma. A solitary, flesh-colored to bluish, cystic lesion about the eyes is characteristic.

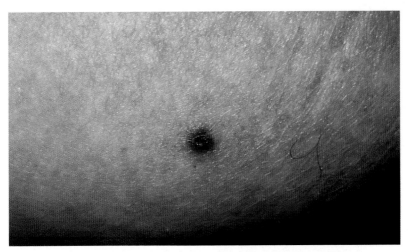

Figure 665. Apocrine hydrocystoma, pigmented.   The fluid secreted into an apocrine hydrocystoma may be so dark blue–black that the lesion may appear nevomelanocytic.

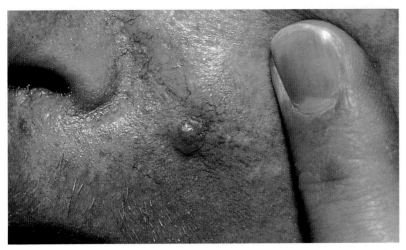

Figure 666. Lymphangioma.   Grouped vesicles with onset from birth to adulthood are characteristic of lymphangioma circumscriptum. Their appearance has been likened to frog spawn. The fluid may be blood-tinged or show a blood–fluid line. These lesions often communicate with deeper lymphatics.

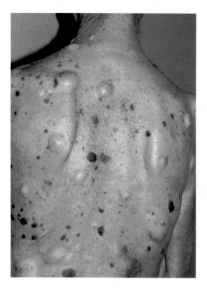

Figure 667. Steatocystoma multiplex.
Multiple, soft, cystic papulonodules develop on the chest, back, axilla, and elsewhere in steatocystoma multiplex. They may range from 2 mm to 4 cm in size. The contents range from milky-white to clear and oily. Rupture, inflammation, and scarring of individual cysts may occur. Inheritance is autosomal dominant.

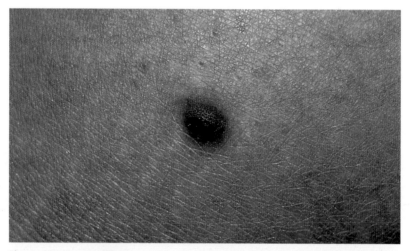

Figure 668. Dermatofibroma.   The patient typically presents with a firm, red, brown, or flesh-colored papule on the leg. The surface may be smooth, hyperkeratotic, or velvety. The upper back and arms are other possible sites. Multiple dermatofibromas (e.g. more than 15) have been associated with various diseases, including lupus erythematosus.

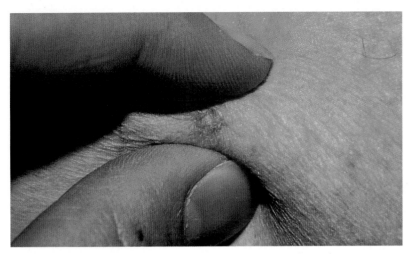

Figure 669. Dermatofibroma, buttonhole sign. Application of lateral pressure causes the center to dimple.

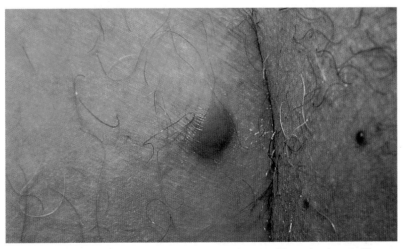

Figure 670. Fibrohistiocytoma. This benign neoplasm is akin to the dermatofibroma but histologically is more cellular with less epidermal change. The patient usually presents with one or more flesh-colored to pink–red firm dermal nodules.

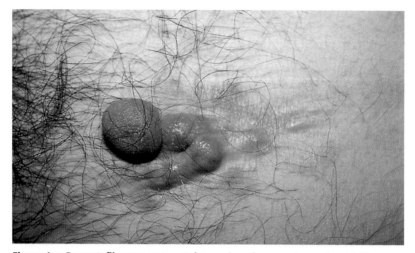

Figure 671. Dermatofibrosarcoma protuberans is a slow-growing malignant fibrous tumor that rarely metastasizes, but may recur locally. A slowly growing firm plaque that later becomes multinodular on the trunk or proximal extremities in an adult is characteristic. Congenital lesions have been reported, and lesions have occurred at sites of a previous trauma e.g. vaccination site, bayonet wound. (Courtesy of Michael O Murphy, MD.)

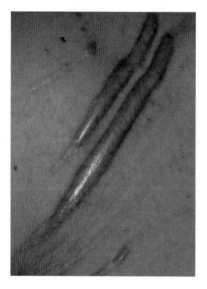

Figure 672. Hypertrophic scar.
An elevated and excessive growth of fibrous tissue within and not extending beyond the bounds of a scar is characteristic. Hypertrophic scars usually resolve over time, whereas keloids usually do not. This patient's hypertrophic scars developed after a motorcycle accident.

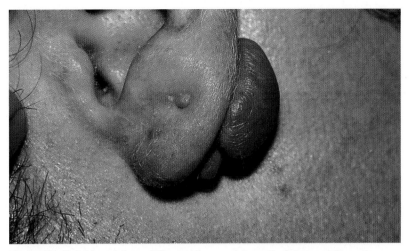

Figure 673. Keloid, earlobe.   A firm, rubbery nodule on the lobe, usually on the posterior surface after ear piercing, is characteristic. Keloids most commonly affect young people of all skin types and dark-skinned people of all ages. Note the two keloids after two ear piercings. Other favored sites include the neck, shoulders, and back.

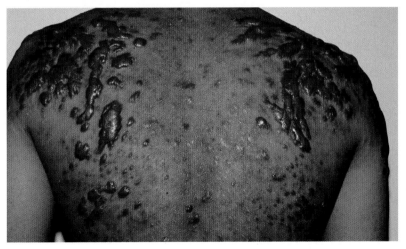

Figure 674. Keloid, diffuse.   The midline of the chest, shoulders, and back are favorite locations for the formation of firm, rubbery, papular or nodular keloids. The pattern of many keloids about the shoulders and upper back is typically caused by severe acne, as is the case for this patient.

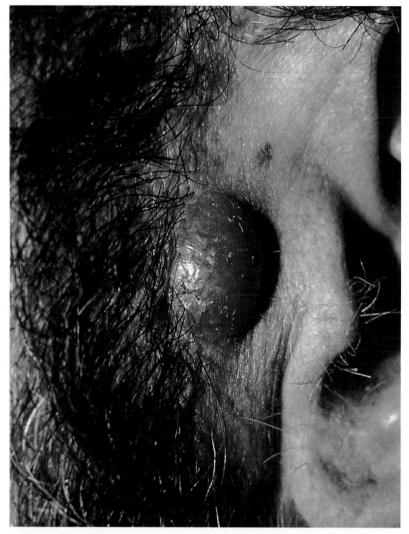

Figure 675. Lymphocytoma cutis.   This nodule represents a dermal collection of inflammatory cells with an abundance of lymphocytes. Clinically, a 0.5–2 cm asymptomatic, erythematous to plum-colored papule or nodule is seen. They may occur virtually anywhere but have a special predilection for the face and ears. A skin biopsy, complete blood count, and lymph node examination are reasonable to help exclude malignancy, e.g. leukemia or lymphoma cutis. In most cases, the cause is not known, but gold exposure (e.g. piercing, acupuncture) or *Borrelia burgdorferi* infection may be associated.

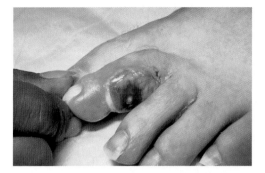

Figure 676. Lymphoma cutis. A lymphoma may rarely present in the skin. Clinically, one sees solitary or multiple, red papulonodules. The clinical differentiation between lymphoma and pseudo-lymphoma may be difficult. (Courtesy of Michael O Murphy, MD.)

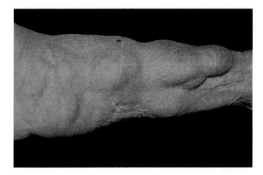

Figure 677. Lipoma, multiple. A lipoma represents a subcutaneous collection of fat. It may be solitary or multiple. The back is a favored site. Unlike an epidermal inclusion cyst, the lipoma has no pore and the overlying skin is movable and unattached to the lesion.

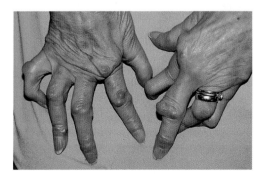

Figure 678. Rheumatoid nodule. Patients with rheumatoid arthritis may develop these nodules over bony prominences such as the knuckles and elbows. These nodules most commonly occur in association with rheumatoid arthritis but may also be seen in systemic lupus erythematosus and scleroderma.

URTICARIAS

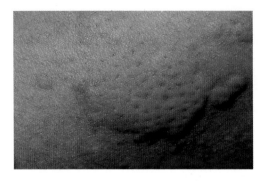

Figure 679. Urticaria. Itchy, edematous, raised, pink plaques without scale that move and change daily are characteristic. Annular lesions resulting from central clearing, and white halos (like the Woronoff's ring of psoriasis) can occur. Delayed pressure urticaria, angioedema, and dermatographism may accompany urticaria.

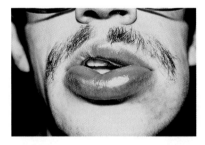

Figure 680. Angioedema is an allergic reaction in which there is significant swelling of tissue, commonly of the lips, eyes, or face. It often accompanies urticaria. If the upper respiratory tract is involved, shortness of breath and even death may occur. Involvement of the GI tract may cause significant abdominal symptoms. Both acquired and inherited forms occur. In hereditary angioedema, patients suffer from periodic attacks of angioedema, nausea, and abdominal and urinary symptoms. Inheritance is autosomal dominant, with several different defects having been found (and mapped to chromosome 11). Each defect results in a deficiency in the proper functioning of the inhibitor of C1. Attacks characterized solely by abdominal symptoms may occur. In fact, many patients undergo abdominal surgery before the proper diagnosis is made. In acquired angioedema, precipitants include allergy to a variety of allergens, including foods and drugs, initiation of ACE inhibitor therapy (thought to cause angioedema by prolonging the effect of bradykinin), and lymphoproliferation and/or antibody directed against the C1 inhibitor. (Courtesy of Michael O Murphy, MD)

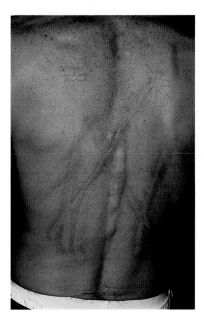

Figure 681. Dermatographism.
Patients with dermatographism may present with the chief complaint of itching. Only rarely will they say, 'My skin turns red and becomes raised wherever I scratch it', although this is exactly what occurs, and is illustrated here. Dermatographism may occur in various clinical situations, including the third trimester of pregnancy or after treatment for scabies. The diagnosis may be established by taking a tongue blade and stroking it several times across the back. Immediate redness will occur in most people, but true whealing will develop within minutes in patients with dermatographism.

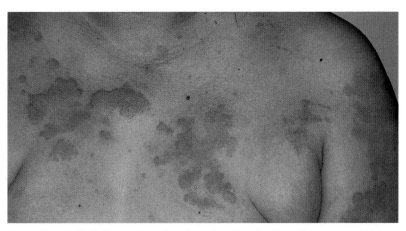

Figure 682. Urticaria is an IgE-mediated reaction. The diet, over-the-counter products, recent illnesses, and medication history should be reviewed for any new potential allergens. If the condition becomes chronic (>6 weeks), laboratory work-up may be performed. (See also **Figure 120**.)

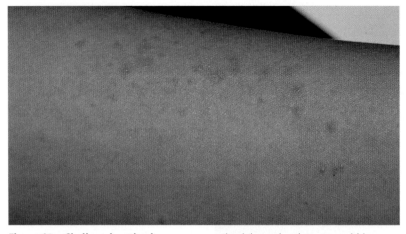

Figure 683. Cholinergic urticaria. 1–4 mm urticarial papules that occur within minutes of exercise are characteristic. The patient can be made to exercise to the point of sweating in the office or just outside to establish the diagnosis.

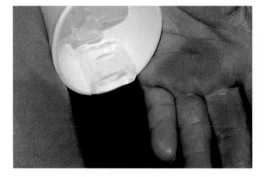

Figure 684. Cold urticaria. Urticarial lesions develop on the fingers after exposure to the cold. Fullness of the throat or swelling of the lips may occur when drinking cold liquids or eating ice cream. Swelling of the head, face and ears may occur after coming indoors from the cold. The ice-cube test is performed as follows: apply two ice cubes to the forearm for 10 minutes. Watch for whealing minutes after removal.

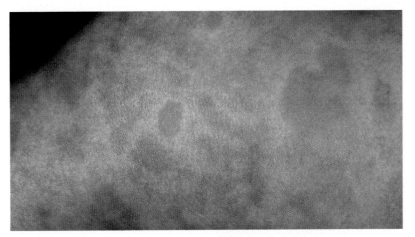

Figure 685. Urticarial vasculitis. Urticarial lesions that last more than 24 hours in any given spot are characteristic. After the initial lesion resolves, purpura remains, as illustrated here. In the acute stage, diascopy will blanch the erythema, allowing visualization of the purpura. Histology shows a leukocytoclastic vasculitis. Urticarial vasculitis is not a specific disease but instead a clinical finding that is usually associated with a vasculitis that causes significant permeability of the dermal microvasculature. Diseases that have been associated or have similar lesions include lupus erythematosus, viral hepatitis, cryoglobulins, and Schnitzler's syndrome. (See also **Figure 123**.)

For related disease, see also solar urticaria (**Figure 476.**)

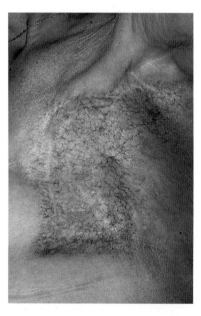

Figure 686. Chronic radiation dermatitis, multiple telangiectases. Years after radiation exposure, the skin becomes indurated and atrophic with mottled pigmentation and telangiectases. This woman's breast cancer radiation port has developed such changes.

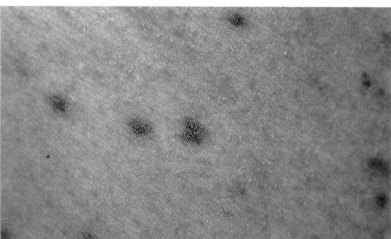

Figure 687. Telangiectasia macularis eruptiva perstans. This variant of mastocytosis presents with telangiectatic macules, often on the trunk of a woman. Special stains (e.g. Giemsa) may be needed to help identify the mast cells histologically. (See also **Figures 18** and **103–105**.)

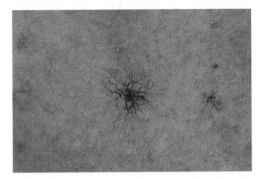

Figure 688. Spider angiomas. An arcade of vessels radiating from a central arteriole produces the characteristic appearance. Compressing the central point blanches the arcade. It is very common in children, in pregnancy, and with liver disease. (See also **Figure 90**.)

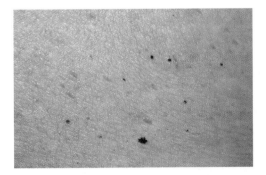

Figure 689. Cherry hemangiomas. Most adults over 30 have one or more red, vascular papules on the trunk. Sometimes, they appear almost 'petechial' as 1–2 mm red macules. In one study of adults 30–39 years of age, 90% of the men and 65% of the women had at least one cherry angioma.

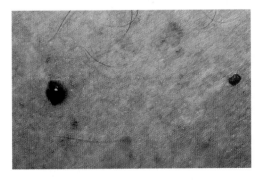

Figure 690. Cherry hemangiomas. The lesion on the right is a true 'cherry' angioma because of its color. The lesion on the left is dark blue because it contains relatively deoxygenated blood.

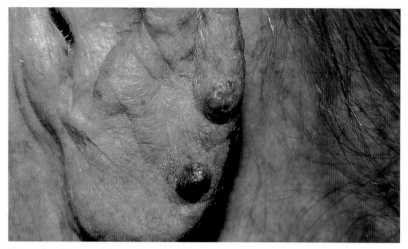

Figure 691. Venous lake.   This dark blue vascular papule that can be completely compressed is common on the lips, ears and face.

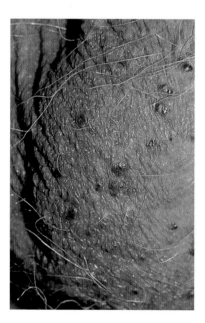

Figure 692. Angiokeratomas, scrotum. Small (1–6 mm), vascular, red papules on the scrotum of an older man are characteristic. They are benign and are usually found incidentally.

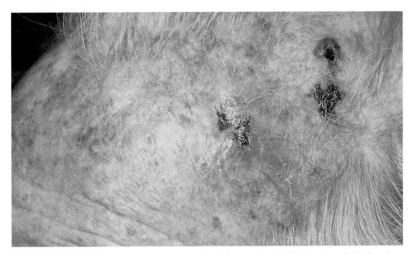

Figure 693. Angiosarcoma of the head and neck. A bruise-like lesion of the head or neck in an elderly patient is characteristic. Vascular papules, nodules or plaques, ulceration and bleeding are common. This highly aggressive vascular tumor may lead to death from local invasion or distant metastases. (Courtesy of Duane Whitaker, MD.)

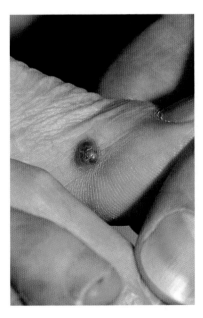

Figure 694. Kaposi's sarcoma, classic type. Kaposi's sarcoma is a vascular proliferation that is related to infection by the human herpes virus 8. The classic type occurs in men of Southern or Eastern European descent. A reddish-blue to purple papulonodule or plaque beginning on the toe or sole is characteristic. Slow progression may occur, with lesions ascending the leg to all parts of the body. Many other organs may be involved but, because of the slow progression of the disease, most patients die of unrelated causes.

For related diseases, see also hereditary hemorrhagic telangiectasia (**Figure 73**) and angiokeratoma, thrombosed (**Figure 485**).

VASCULOPATHIES

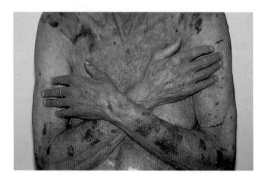

Figure 695. Purpura secondary to topical corticosteroids. Chronic use of topical steroids can result in thinning of the skin, purpura, and stretch marks. This older patient had used clobetasol propionate for several months to control his subacute cutaneous lupus erythematosus.

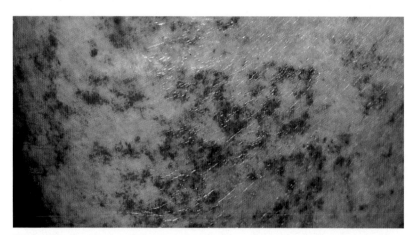

Figure 696. Progressive pigmentary dermatosis. The sudden appearance on the lower legs of many bright red petechiae is characteristic. Some have likened the appearance to Cayenne pepper. Later, the lesions turn brown. The underlying process is a capillaritis, resulting in extravasation of blood. Most often, no cause is found, although a new drug or vitamin may be implicated.

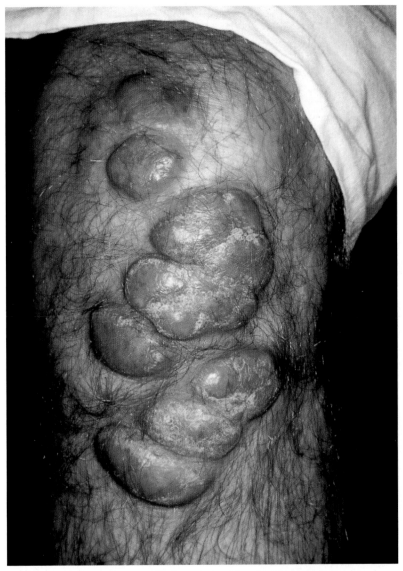

Figure 697. Erythema elevatum diutinum is considered a rare variant of leukocytoclastic vasculitis that leads to fibrosis and deposition of lipid. Although chronic, there is no systemic vasculopathy, although arthralgias may be present. A monoclonal gammopathy (particularly IgA but also IgG), myeloma (particularly IgA myeloma), and hypergammaglobulinemia have also been associated. This disease has been associated with a variety of other diseases, including hematologic malignancies, infections, etc. Red–brown nodules are found symmetrically on the dorsa of the hands, elbows, and knees. (Courtesy of Gary Cole, MD.)

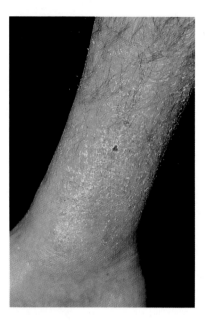

Figure 698. Stasis dermatitis. A red, scaly rash over the medial part of the ankle associated with pitting edema in an older, often overweight, individual is characteristic. The entire lower leg may be involved. Severe edema may lead to beads of fluid and bulla formation. In later stages, the skin may develop a red–brown hue secondary to hemosiderin deposition. Allergic contact dermatitis to topical medication may complicate the clinical picture.

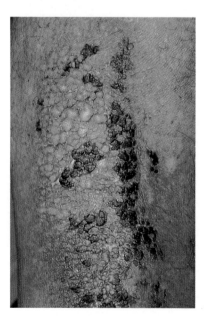

Figure 699. Elephantiasis verruciformis nostra. A chronically enlarged, edematous leg or legs with a verrucous or cobble-stoned surface is characteristic. Stemmer's sign (thickening of the skin over the dorsal toes or fingers) is an early change. Recurrent cellulitis is a frequent finding. The disease results from blockage of the lymphatics (e.g. by venous stasis, malignancy). Elephantiasis of the legs, scrotum, penis, and vulva may occur in some parts of the world from lymphatic obstruction by filaria.

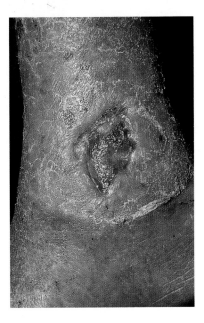

Figure 700. Venous ulcer. Venous ulceration may occur in the setting of chronic stasis. An X-ray to rule out osteomyelitis or a biopsy to rule out malignancy may be indicated for prolonged ulcers. Osteoarthritis, stroke, rheumatoid arthritis, or obesity are common contributory factors.

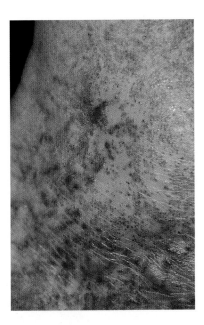

Figure 701. Atrophie blanche. Smooth, white, stellate plaques about the ankle and foot in a woman with chronic venous insufficiency are characteristic of atrophie blanche. The initial lesion is often a purpuric papule or a hemorrhagic bulla followed by a painful ulcer. The stellate, white scar results on healing.

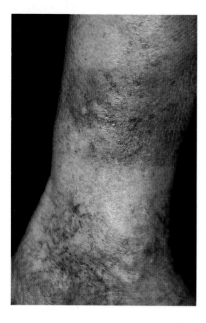

Figure 702. Lipodermatosclerosis.
Also known as sclerosing panniculitis, lipodermatosclerosis manifests itself as an indurated, adherent, erythematous, well-defined area on the medial aspect of the lower leg in the setting of chronic venous insufficiency. The lesion may be elevated, flat or depressed. A biopsy should be avoided if possible, as healing will invariably be difficult.
In this figure, the red plaque represents lipodermatosclerosis. Ankle flare and atrophie blanche are seen on the medial ankle.

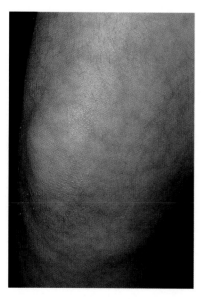

Figure 703. Cutis marmorata.
A reticulated or mottled appearance of the skin in response to cold is characteristic. It is common in infants but may affect all ages. It is entirely benign and may be considered a variant of normal.

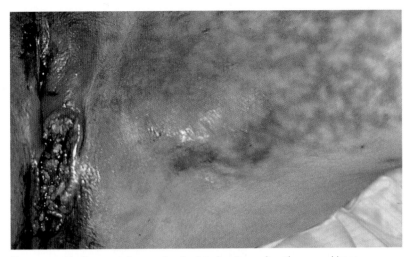

Figure 704. Erythema ab igne. A reticulated pattern of erythema and later hyperpigmentation at the site of chronic thermal exposure (e.g. from a heater, heating pad, fire) is characteristic. The thermal damage preferentially occurs in the border areas between the blood-dispersing arterial zones because the heat dispersion in these areas is low. This 41-year-old woman also has a squamous cell carcinoma arising from the anus. (Courtesy of Paul Koonings, MD.)

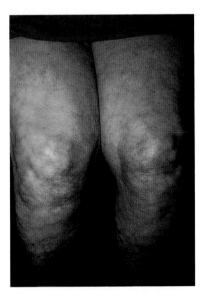

Figure 705. Livedo reticularis. A reticulated, blanching, vascular pattern of the legs occurs as a cutaneous sign of underlying vascular obstructive disease in livedo reticularis. The general work-up should include taking a history (recent infection, drug ingestion, history of cerebrovascular accident or hypertension), a biopsy deep enough to sample medium and large arteries, antinuclear antibody, rheumatoid factor, erythrocyte sedimentation rate, anticardiolipin antibody (positive in this case), antineutrophil cytoplasmic antibody, cryoglobulins, complete blood count, and renal and hepatic blood tests.

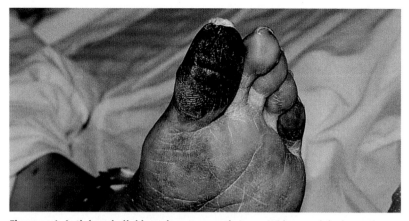

Figure 706. Antiphospholipid syndrome, necrotic toe.   Widespread dusky erythema, cutaneous necrosis, leg ulceration, livedo reticularis, splinter hemorrhages, and ecchymosis all occur in the antiphospholipid syndrome. The diagnosis requires that a patient has recurrent thrombosis (e.g. deep vein thrombosis, pulmonary emboli, cerebral infarction) or fetal loss (e.g. abortion, intrauterine death), and a positive antiphospholipid antibody. The disease may be primary or secondary (occurring in association with other diseases, the classic being systemic lupus erythematosus) or as a familial trait.

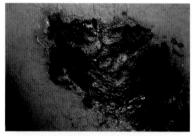

Figure 707. Coumadin necrosis.
Necrosis of the skin 3–6 days after starting warfarin or 3–6 days after excessive hypocoagulability in a patient receiving warfarin is characteristic. The skin is initially painful and edematous, followed by ecchymosis, hemorrhagic bullae, and necrosis. The presumed mechanism is via the more rapid initial decrease in the protein C anticoagulant activity compared with the slower decline of other vitamin-K-dependent factors.

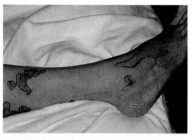

Figure 708. Disseminated intravascular coagulation.   Widespread areas of necrosis in a patient who is profoundly ill are characteristic. The loss of normal inhibition of clotting mechanisms leads to intravascular coagulation associated with consumption of platelets and clotting factors. Associated/underlying diseases include Gram-negative sepsis and shock. The skin marks seen here help to monitor progression.

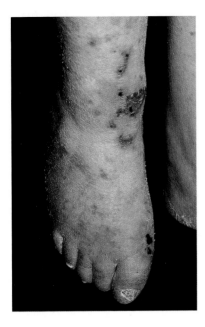

Figure 709. Cholesterol emboli is a condition in which particles from the inner wall of larger blood vessels embolize to extremities, causing impaired blood supply to the skin. Often patients have a history of a prior arteriography, although arteriography may help localize a source. Usually the onset is within hours or days of the procedure, although 3 cases with onset of symptoms 5–16 weeks after undergoing a vascular procedure have been reported. Common manifestations include livedo reticularis, gangrene, cyanosis, ulceration, nodules, and purpura. Diagnosis may be confirmed by finding cholesterol crystal clefts in the dermal blood vessels.

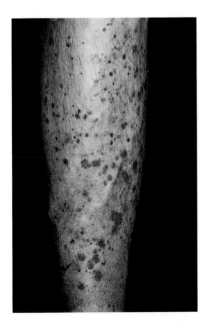

Figure 710. Palpable purpura. Leukocytoclastic vasculitis is a histologic description of a type of small vessel vasculitis. Clinically, one sees a shower of purpuric lesions, both palpable and non-palpable, concentrated on the legs. (For further discussion, see **Figure 244.**)

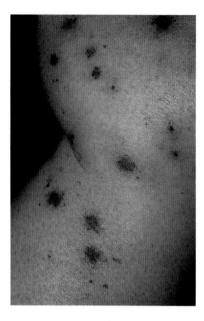

Figure 711. Hypersensitivity vasculitis from a medication. Hypersensitivity to a medication can precipitate a cutaneous small vessel vasculitis, e.g. leukocytoclastic vasculitis. Other terms for hypersensitivity vasculitis are necrotizing vasculitis and allergic angiitis. (See also **Figure 244**.)

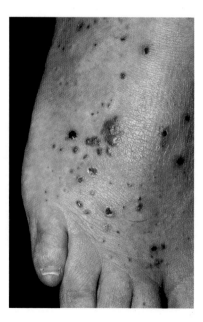

Figure 712. Henoch–Schönlein purpura, adult. Henoch–Schönlein purpura may occur in adults. When the skin is involved, it may present with palpable purpura, as shown here. The pathogenesis involves deposition of immune complexes in which most of the antibody is of the IgA class. A variety of target antigens may be involved (e.g. infectious agents). (See also **Figure 126**.)

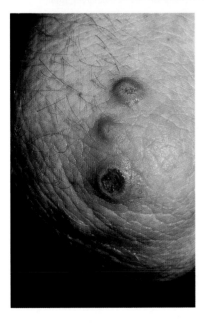

Figure 713. Rheumatoid vasculitis is an uncommon manifestation of rheumatoid arthritis. Clinical features may range from an indolent skin disease (e.g. nailfold infarcts, petechiae, and livedo reticularis) to a life-threatening multi-organ vasculitis resembling polyarteritis nodosa (e.g. with necrotic ulcers, digital gangrene, and mononeuritis multiplex). The rheumatoid factor is usually high.

Figure 714. Wegener's granulomatosis. The triad of necrotizing granulomatous vasculitis of the upper and lower respiratory tracts, glomerulonephritis, and small vessel vasculitis characterizes Wegener's granulomatosis. The average age of onset is middle age, with skin lesions occurring in about a quarter of patients. Cutaneous lesions include palpable purpura, hemorrhagic or necrotic papulonodules, pustules, erosions, bullae, and ulcers. The lower leg is most commonly affected. A distinctive gingivitis (granular with petechiae) occurs. Oral ulcers are characteristic and are persistent, in contrast to aphthous ulcers. Cutaneous ulcers sometimes resemble pyoderma gangrenosum and may exhibit pathergy. They usually lack the raised, tender, undermined border, however. Subglottic stenosis and nasal deformity are much more common in childhood cases. The criteria for diagnosis include nasal or oral inflammation (e.g. nasal discharge, oral ulcers), an abnormal CXR, an abnormal urine sediment, granulomatous inflammation on biopsy, and a positive c-ANCA. The antineutrophil cytoplasmic antibody is characteristic and is positive in approximately 85–100% of patients with active disease.

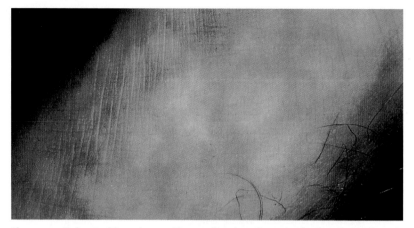

Figure 715. Polyarteritis nodosa. The small and medium-sized arteries are affected by a necrotizing vasculitis which leads to palpable purpura, punched out ulcers, tender subcutaneous nodules, and livedo reticularis (shown here). Fever, malaise, myalgias, arthralgias, arthritis, cardiac insufficiency, renal aneurysms, and polyneuropathy may occur. A related and possibly causative antigen should be sought, e.g. hepatitis B, HIV, and, in children, recent streptococcal infection. (Courtesy of James Rasmussen, MD.)

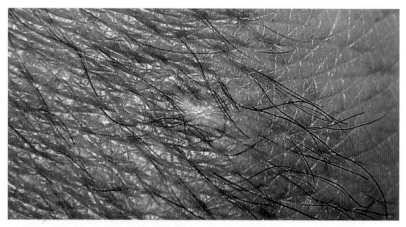

Figure 716. Malignant atrophic papulosis (Dego's disease) is a rare, often fatal disorder characterized by multiple infarcts in the skin and internal organs. The underlying cause is a thrombotic vasculopathy of unknown origin. Erythematous papules on the trunk and proximal extremities that develop into atrophic, white, porcelain-centered lesions in a young to middle-aged man are characteristic. A wedge-shaped area of necrosis is seen histologically in this disease. The gastrointestinal tract is the second most commonly involved organ, especially the small intestine.

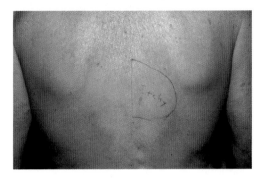

Figure 717. Notalgia paresthetica is a term used to describe a chronic, fixed itch of the back. It is thought to represent a sensory neuropathy of the cutaneous nerves as they take a right angle in their course to that location. Middle-aged to elderly patients may present with a very pruritic, fixed spot on the back just to one side of the midline. Hyperpigmentation may be present and in most patients is thought to be secondary to chronic scratching.

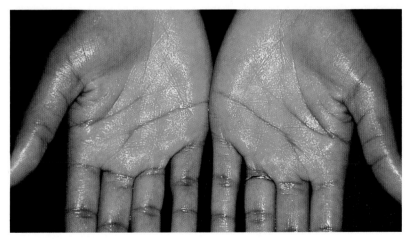

Figure 718. Hyperhidrosis. Excessive sweating of the axilla, palms, and soles occurs in hyperhidrosis. For some reason, patients often do not believe there is treatment for this disease and thus do not seek medical attention. The doctor may notice the condition when shaking hands with the patient who is being seen for another reason. Often patients will carry around a tissue or paper towel and dry their hands just before shaking.

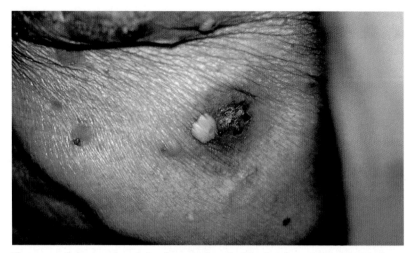

Figure 719. Subcorneal pustular dermatosis. In this chronic pustular dermatosis, also known as Sneddon–Wilkinson disease, sterile superficial pustules develop with a preference for the trunk, axillae, and the flexor aspect of the limbs. Annular lesions occur. A direct immunofluorescence should be obtained (and found negative) to exclude intraepidermal neutrophilic IgA dermatosis. (Courtesy of Gary Cole, MD.)

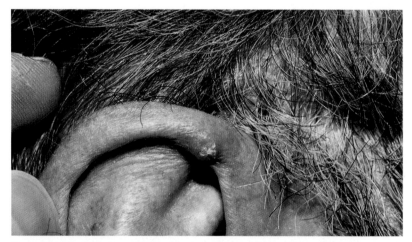

Figure 720. Chondrodermatitis nodularis helices. This painful nodule on the ear of an adult has been called an 'ear corn' and represents inflammation of the cartilage after prolonged pressure. A painful, hyperkeratotic papule on the ear, most often just inferior to Darwin's tubercle in an older man, is characteristic. These lesions may also occur in women and on the antihelix. Habits which exert prolonged pressure on the ear (e.g. sleeping on that side, head phones) help trigger the condition.

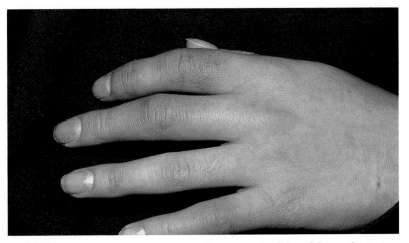

Figure 721. Perniosis, or chilblains, is an inflammatory condition of the acral areas chronically exposed to cold, damp environments. Pruritic, often painful, areas are seen on the fingers and toes. Spontaneous resolution occurs if the areas are kept away from the cold.

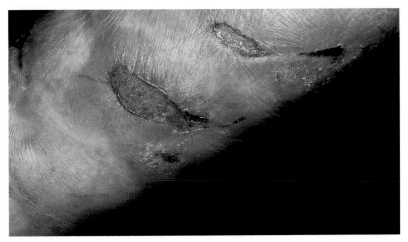

Figure 722. Dermatitis artefacta. Patients with dermatitis artefacta induce their own skin lesions. Diagnosis can be difficult as the clinician must exclude other skin conditions. Ulcers, excoriations, crust, and finally white scars are seen. Self-induced (factitious) skin lesions typically have sharply defined edges and linear or geographic shapes. Lesions always occur in skin accessible to the patient (e.g. not the center of the back). The extensor surfaces are particularly favored. Secondary bacterial infection is common, and thus a bacterial folliculitis may coexist.

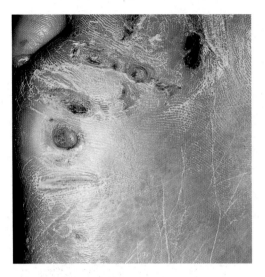

Figure 723. Mal perforans ulcer. This is an ulcer formed after repeated trauma to a pressure area of the sole in the setting of decreased sensation. The typical location is an ulcer over the 1st or 5th metatarsal on the plantar aspect of the foot. The patient is often a diabetic with peripheral neuropathy.

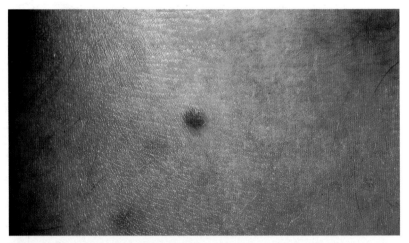

Figure 724. Lymphomatoid papulosis (LP) represents a clonal proliferation of T-cells in the skin, causing papular lesions. A percentage of patients go on to develop systemic lymphoma (e.g. CTCL, Hodgkin's disease, immunoblastic lymphoma, anaplastic large cell lymphoma). One study found that the mean time from onset to the development of lymphoma was 12 years, and that the cumulative risk of developing lymphoma is 80% in patients who have LP for 15 years. This has led some experts to consider LP a low-grade malignant CTCL. Some cases are borderline between LP and CD30 (Ki-1)-positive large cell lymphoma. The initial lesion is an erythematous to red/brown papule (as shown) which in days to weeks may become hemorrhagic or necrotic. Multiple, self-healing lesions occurring in crops in an adult are characteristic. The disease may last from weeks to decades.

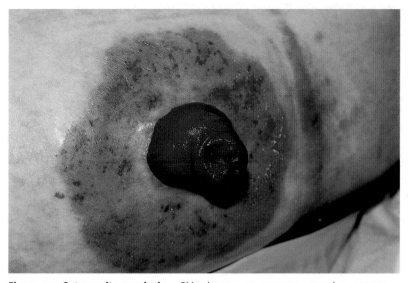

Figure 725. Ostomy site, psoriasis. Skin changes are common around an ostomy site. Leakage may occur leading to an irritant dermatitis. Intertrigo may develop from sweating, maceration, and increased friction. Bacterial infection signaled by pustules or erosion may occur. A red, scaly rash may indicate a fungal infection. Allergic contact dermatitis manifested as an eczematous rash may occur and can be ruled in or out by appliance use on the contralateral side. Encrustations and pseudoepitheliomatous hyperplasia occur. Rarely, periostomal pyoderma gangrenosum may develop (see **Figure 420**). Finally, any skin condition that Köbnerizes (occurs at sites of trauma) may affect the ostomy site. A patient with psoriasis is shown.

INDEX

B